MW01258730

For God
and
Country

Operation Whitecoat: 1954–1973

By

Commander Robert L. Mole
Chaplain Corps
United States Navy (Retired)

and

Commander Dale M. Mole
Medical Corps
United States Navy

TEACH Services, Inc
Brushton, New York

PRINTED IN THE UNITED STATES OF AMERICA
World rights reserved. This book or any portion thereof may not
be copied or reproduced in any form or manner whatever,
except as provided by law, without the written permission of the
publisher, except by a reviewer who may quote brief passages
in a review.

The authors assume full responsibility for the accuracy of all facts
and quotations as cited in this book. The opinions or assertions
herein are those of the authors and are not to be construed as
official or as reflecting the views of the U.S. Navy, Department of
Defense, Government of the United States of America, or the
Seventh-day Adventist Church.

Copyright © 1998 Dale Mole

ISBN 1–57258–138–7
Library of Congress Catalog Card No. 98–86442

Published by

TEACH Services, Inc.
254 Donovan Road
Brushton, New York 12916–9738

It is not the critic who counts, nor the man who points out how the strong man stumbled, or where the doer of the deed could have done better. The credit belongs to the man who is actually in the arena; whose face is marred by dust and sweat and blood; who survives valiantly; who errs and comes short again and again; who knows great enthusiasms, great devotions, who spends himself in a worthy cause; who, at the best, knows in the end the triumph of high achievement; and who, at the worst, if he fails, at least fails while daring greatly, so that his place shall never be with those cold and timid souls who know neither victory nor defeat.

Theodore Roosevelt

Table of Contents

IN MEMORIUM

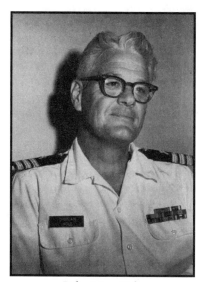

Robert Lee Mole
1923–1993

How does one sum up an exceptional life of three score and ten years in a few short sentences? He was a Christian, Minister, Missionary, Patriot, Scholar, Teacher, Anthropologist, Warrior, Son, Brother, Husband, Father, Friend, Comforter, Pioneer, Author, Sailor, and Master Gardener.

Born in 1923 on a dairy farm in Florida, a product of the great Depression, a self-made man, he was known as a practical person with a great thirst for knowledge. Never knowing a stranger, he befriended all. His home was open to everyone who cared to partake of "rusty water and moldy bread."

After serving as a missionary in the Middle East, he returned home to become the first Seventh-day Adventist chaplain in the United States Navy. He survived two tours in Vietnam and was awarded the Bronze Star with a 'V' attachment for valor; one of his twelve medals and decorations. He served his country for twenty-three years in uniform, his last tour was at Arlington National Cemetery where he referred to himself as the "Virginia Planter." He then went on to serve as a chaplain in the Veterans Administration hospital system until his death.

Always a professional student, he earned a Master of Arts in Religion from the Seventh-day Adventist Theological Seminary, Washington, D.C. in 1946, a Master of Arts in Divinity from the same institution in 1957, a Master of Arts in Clinical Education from the Lutheran School of Theology, Chicago, in 1963, a Master of Arts in Area Studies from American University in 1970, a Master of Arts in Religion and Medical Care from George Washington University in 1972, and a Doctor of Sacred Ministry from Howard University School of Religion in 1974.

My father was a special person in my life. Judging from the number of people who told me how he had made a difference in their lives, he was obviously very special to many others. We miss you Dad.

Dale Michael Mole
Virginia Beach, VA

DEDICATION

Operation Whitecoat: for God and Country, is dedicated to General W.D. Tigertt, M.D., U.S. Army; and to Colonel Dan Crozier, M.D., U.S. Army and to Doctor and Mrs. Frank S. Damazo, M.D., of Frederick, Maryland.

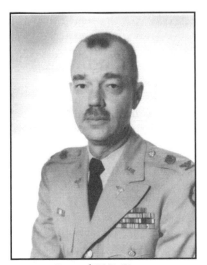

General W.D. Tigertt

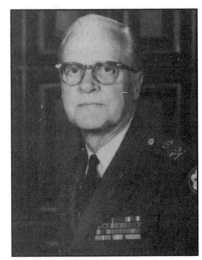

Colonel Dan Crozier

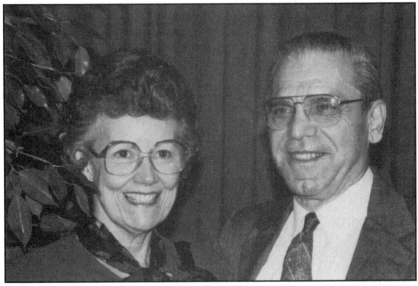

Dr. & Mrs. Frank Damazo

Doctor Damazo served in the Army Medical Corps from April 1951 to May 1953 as a surgeon in Japan for American casualties of the Korean War, as well as a year in Korea as a physician for the Korean and Chinese prisoners of war. While in the Far East, he experienced and enjoyed the hospitality of Doctor and Mrs. George Rue, Pastor and Mrs. Paul Nelson, and Pastor and Mrs. Verne Kalstrom. Their Sabbath services, meals, and moral support for servicemen paid rich dividends, as the Damazos, with the Frederick, Maryland Seventh-day Adventist Church, have carried on this tradition at the U.S. Army's Fort Detrick. As a practicing general surgeon in Frederick, Maryland, Doctor Damazo has continued to maintain a positive relationship with the United States Army Medical Research Institute of Infectious Diseases (USAMRIID). His personal contacts with USAMRIID have been very valuable in gathering information for this volume.

Doctor Damazo and his wife are unique in that their concern and interest in Operation Whitecoat has continued over the years, from its beginning in 1954 to the present. Their involvement has included not only financial support in numerous unpublicized ways, but they also have been the primary personalities in ongoing Whitecoat reunions. Their interest also includes strong encouragement to have the story of Operation Whitecoat related in a dispassionate, factual style so that a double purpose may be fulfilled. First, to tell of men willing to be human subjects in experimental medical research which have resulted in findings that greatly reduce human suffering and death, and secondly, so the lessons learned might provide moral and ethical guidelines should the need for other such medical studies arise in the future.

General W.D. Tigertt, M.D. was a key player in Operation Whitecoat, as he was the senior Army physician in the initial and ongoing relations with the General Conference of Seventh-day Adventists from 1954 until his retirement in 1961. The dream he personified and the rapport he fostered with the Seventh-day Adventist Church continued until the operation ended in 1972 following the suspension of the military draft. His openness in explaining the goals and procedures, as well as the inherent principles, of Operation Whitecoat did much to enable the General Conference to believe this medical research was in harmony with its theology and understanding of biblical truth.

Colonel Dan Crozier, M.D. was a giant among men as a physician, military officer, and medical scientist. Beyond all of these accomplishments has been his sense of mission and concern for those within his Command. His willingness to personally be injected with every vaccine before its use on Whitecoat volunteers, as well as his personal openness, endeared him to his patients and his peers.

It would be an injustice not to recognize and gratefully acknowledge the work of SP/5 Errol L. Chamness, U.S. Army, whose historical efforts have proven invaluable. Also special mention needs to be made of Colonel Arthur Anderson, MC, USA for his assistance in providing information regarding current USAMRIID activities. USAMRIID cooperated in the research of this volume by sharing its archives, reviewing the manuscript in its formative stages, and assuring that significant information has been made available. Special appreciation and recognition is given to Mr. Norman Corvert, Historian and Public Affairs Officer at Fort Detrick, Maryland, and his able assistant Eileen Mitchel, for their support, information, photographs and cooperation. Their assistance was vital in bringing to light, important but often difficult to find, details of Opertion Whitecoat.

For critical review of the manuscript, suggestions regarding form and content, as well as general support and encouragement, sincere thanks must be extended to the helpful staff at Adventist Chaplaincy Ministries, including Dick Stenbakken, Martin Feldbush, Rachel Child, and Linda Mercer.

Sincerest appreciation must be expressed to Chaplain Mole's secretaries, Nancy Cannon and Deborah Loar, for their personal dedication and efforts in the preparation of this book. Roberta Lee Mole Booth proofread parts of the final manuscript. Dolores S. Kinsey assisted in editing parts of the original manuscript.

Lastly, it would be remiss not to include in the dedication of this volume the nearly three thousand American military conscientious objector noncombatants (1–A–O) who volunteered, whatever their rationales, to be utilized as subjects in experimental medical research, primarily in airborne infectious diseases. Their story should be told so their children and others may know of and appreciate the men who were willing to risk their lives, not on the battlefields of tanks, planes, bombs, and bullets, but in the quiet laboratories where the battle against deadly diseases continues, unabated in war or peace.

FORWARD

The Johns Hopkins University
School of Hygiene and Public Health
Department of Immunology & Infectious Diseases

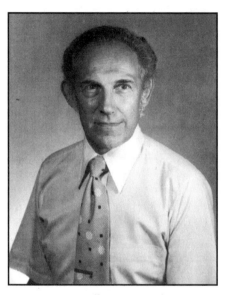

Dr. William R. Beisel

Much has been said about the military value of the Whitecoat Program and its moral/ethical aspects. As a physician/research scientist, I would like to mention the extremely valuable scientific contributions to medical knowledge that arose from the Whitecoat Program. These contributions were important to military medical knowledge, to be sure. But other extraordinary contributions to worldwide medical progress, made possible ONLY by the Whitecoat Program, proved to be even more valuable, in my mind. These additional contributions to medical knowledge were a quite unexpected bonus of the Program, because they provided medical information that remains current today, helping physicians throughout the world to treat problems involved with infectious diseases, starvation, and stresses of many varieties.

Before the Whitecoat Program, physicians could only begin studying infections when they first saw a patient, usually one or more days after fever had begun. But with the Whitecoats, normal baseline data could be gathered before exposure,…plus daily measurements throughout the incubation period, before fever began. To this new examination of the onset of infection were added the metabolic, endocrine, and physiologic studies that were superimposed on the vaccine evaluation protocols. Such broad studies had never been done previously. Although such studies caused the Whitecoat volunteers to endure weeks of feeding only on soy milkshake diets, or weeks of eight hours-a-day toil on computer consoles, or semi-starvation, or 24 hours of exposure in a steam-filled hot room, the data that emerged have everlasting medical worth.

The medical information on losses of body nutrients and biochemical and metabolic changes during infection has proven to be of vast importance in attempting to cure infections in malnourished patients, especially infants and small children, and the aged. The combination of infection and malnutrition kills more people throughout the world, thousands every day, than any other disease. The same information has also proven valuable in treating patients with severe medical or surgical diseases.

These studies of Whitecoats provided the first prospective information about hormonal changes during infection, changes that involved pituitary, adrenal, thyroid, and pancreatic hormones. Subsequently, many scientists throughout the world have detected similar changes in many different forms of stress. Similar endocrine changes have recently been observed during U.S. Army Ranger training. All these stress-related data are now under current review and study by the National Academy of Science.

The Whitecoat data was republished in 1991 in the 2nd Edition of a major textbook, *Nutritional Biochemistry and Metabolism*. The data is also republished as the first chapter of the 3rd Edition of Ralph Feigin's huge, two volume, textbook, *Pediatric Infectious Disease*. Dr. Feigin, now head of Pediatrics and the Children's Hospital of Baylor University, was once one of the USAMRIID research physicians who worked with me in Whitecoat studies. I continue to use the data in all the courses I teach. I cannot say the number of times I have blessed the Whitecoat volunteers for their bravery and dedication in contributing themselves to these studies.

William R. Beisel, M.D., F.A.C.P., Adjunct Professor
Baltimore, Maryland

A SHORT HISTORY OF BIOLOGICAL WARFARE

Down through the ages, infectious disease has played a major role in shaping the course of world events. Great civilizations were altered or extinguished merely from exposure to microscopic organisms. What was true in the past is true today. The war against infectious disease continues. Few realize that every day brings the death of approximately forty thousand children, the majority from infectious disease.

Infectious disease has also played a significant role in the success or failure of many military campaigns. Far more brave warriors were lost to the ravages of the invisible microbe than were felled by the well aimed stone, sword blow, arrow, musket ball, or high velocity rifle bullet. As one attempts to gain advantage over a more powerful and well-equipped enemy, the intentional dissemination of disease adds a new dimension to threat of disease acquired by natural means.

The use of biological agents as weapons of war and terrorism date back many centuries. As early as the 6th century BC, the Assyrians attempted to incapacitate their enemies by clandestinely poisoning their wells with rye ergot, a known hallucinogen. During the same time period, the Solon warriors used the purgative herb hellebore to induce explosive diarrhea in the inhabitants of Krissa, during a siege of the city.

In 400 B.C., Scythian archers dipped their arrowheads in blood and manure or decomposing bodies in an effort to increase the lethality of their weapons. As one of the first reported Naval uses of biological agents, Hannibal is reported to have hurled venomous snakes onto the enemy vessels of Pergamus at Eurymedon in 190 B.C.

Leaping forward to the middle ages, the practice of placing dead bodies in a enemy's water supply proved to be an effective means of inducing disease, as demonstrated by Barbarossa in 1155 at the battle of Tortona.

In 1346, plague broke out amongst the Tartar army during it's siege of Kaffa. Seeking to profit from this misfortune, someone developed the gruesome plan of hurling the diseased corpses of dead soldiers over the walls of the city with the hope of infecting the inhabitants. This achieved the desired effect and resulting epidemic forced the defenders to surrender.

One of the more imaginative biological weapons was developed by a Polish artillery general named Siemenowics around 1650. Searching for an unpleasant means to kill the enemy, he decided to fill his hollow artillery rounds with saliva from rabid dogs. The success of this weapon was never recorded, but one could imagine it's effect psychologically.

The scourge of smallpox (variola) was successfully employed by the Europeans during their conquest of the New World. Pizarro is said to have presented South American natives with variola-contaminated clothing in the 15th century. In 1763, Colonel Henry Bouguet, a British officer, suggested giving smallpox infected blankets to the Frankophile Indians at Fort Pitt, Pennsylvania during the French and Indian War.

The American Civil War served as an horrific harbinger of things to come and many new forms of combat were successfully introduced or improved upon; aerial warfare (observation balloons), trench warfare (foreshadowed the battlefields of World War I), and submarine warfare (the first successful submarine attack against a surface ship), just to name a few. Biological warfare in one form or another was also utilized.

In 1861, advancing Union troops were warned not to eat or drink anything provided by unknown civilians in southern Maryland for fear of deliberate adulteration. Despite this warning, there were numerous cases of poisoning. In Mississippi in 1863, hastily retreating Confederate troops left dead animals in wells and ponds to deny water to the enemy. Dr. Luke Blackburn, the future governor of Kentucky, deliberately sold smallpox infected clothing to unsuspecting Union troops.

Humans have not been the exclusive targets of biological warfare. During World War I, German agents infected the Rumanian calvary with glanders, a chronic and debilitating disease that attacks the mucous membranes in nostrils of horses. Once infected, the horses developed copious mucus secretions, accompanied by enlargement of the lymph nodes of the lower jaw.

Even in the United States, a neutral country in the early stages of World War I, agents of the German Empire were active. One clever saboteur, a German naval officer by the name of Captain Erich von Steinmetz, entered the United States disguised as a woman. He carried a culture of glanders, with which he hoped to infect livestock destined for the western front in Europe. When the desired result was not obtained, he took the cultures to a laboratory only to discover they were dead.

A somewhat more successful escapade was engineered by an American-educated surgeon. Dr. Anton Dilger specialized in wound surgery while studying at the Johns Hopkins University in

Baltimore, Maryland. Since his medical skills were in great demand in his home country, Dr. Dilger joined the Germany army in 1914. The war proved to be a bit too much for the good doctor. He soon suffered a nervous breakdown and returned to his parents' home in Virginia to recuperate. Amazingly he obtained permission from the United States government to import strains of anthrax and glanders, supposedly to begin a horse inoculation program. However, he and his brother, Carl, had a hidden agenda. Together they set up "Tony's Lab" in a private house in Chevy Chase, Maryland and began producing bacteria. They then gave the bacteria to Captain Frederick Hinsch, who was living nearby in the port city of Baltimore. Captain Hinsch was able to successfully infect many Europe bound horses.

Natural disease, rather than manmade, was to have a more profound effect upon the American landscape during the Autumn of 1918. A devastating influenza epidemic swept across the countryside. War propagandists accused the Germans of responsibility for instigating the tragedy. While this was later shown to be absurd, mass draft registrations, as well as crowded conditions in military camps and aboard troop ships did much to further the disease's deadly spread.

The effects were profound for both civilian and military populations. During October alone, almost 200,000 Americans died as a result of influenza. During the 10 month epidemic, the death toll reached half a million. This naturally acquired illness well illustrates the extent to which military conflict and infectious disease are intertwined. The need to supply American troops to the battlefields of France overrode President Wilson's concern for quarantine and other preventive measures against this deadly epidemic.

Unfortunately, the "war to end all wars" was not the last major conflict fought in this century. In less than two decades the world was preparing for another conflagration. In 1937, Japan built the infamous biological warfare laboratory, code named "Unit 731," 40 miles south of Harbin, Manchuria. General Ishii directed the ambitious program, using thousands of Chinese nationals as unwilling experimental subjects. Over 3000 prisoners died after being deliberately exposed to anthrax, syphilis, plague, and cholera during a study of the natural (untreated) course of these diseases. Almost 1000 autopsies were performed on victims exposed to aerosolized anthrax alone. By 1945, the Japanese were said to have stockpiled 400 kilograms of anthrax to be used in specially designed bombs. There is evidence Japanese planes dropped plague infected fleas over areas in China and Manchuria, causing epidemics of the disease.

In 1943, the United States began biological warfare research after concern arose regarding a perceived threat from Nazi Germany. With the advent of the V-1 "buzz bomb," the ancestor of the modern cruise missile, the Germans possessed an ideal means by which to disperse deadly aerosols of infective agents over large areas. The United States established a research complex at a small National Guard airfield, known at the time as Detrick Field, in Frederick, Maryland.

Detrick Field, named for an Army flight surgeon, later became Camp Detrick during World War II, then Fort Detrick when it was viewed as a permanent facility. Biological studies included basic science research on infectious agents, methods of delivery, medical treatment, vaccine development, and protective garments.

President Nixon halted all offensive biological weapon research and production by an executive order in 1969. All stockpiles of biologic agents were destroyed in the presence of monitors from the United States Department of Agriculture, the Department of Health, Education, and Welfare, and the states of Arkansas, Colorado, and Maryland between May 1971 and May 1972. The medical defensive program continues today.

In 1972, the Convention on the Prohibition of the Development, Production and Stockpiling of Bacteriological (Biological) and Toxin Weapons, fortunately known by it's shorter name, the Biological Weapons Treaty, was signed into being. Among the many signatories to this accord were the United States, the Soviet Union, and the government of Iraq. Unfortunately, there is clear evidence that several countries have violated this treaty. Among the most widely publicized were the "yellow rain" incidents in Southeast Asia, the accidental release of anthrax at Sverdlovsk, and the use of ricin as an assassination weapon in the 1970's.

Eyewitnesses from the countries of Laos (1975–1981), Kampuchea (1979–1981), and Afghanistan (1979–1981) reported that aircraft-delivered aerosols of several different colors which produced disorientation, generalized illness, and some deaths amongst exposed people and animals. These clouds were thought to contain T2 mycotoxin, and the incidents were named "yellow rain" after the predominate color of the tricholthecene toxin. It has been estimated there were 6,300 deaths in Laos, 1,000 deaths in Kampuchea, and 3,042 deaths in Afghanistan. The victims were usually unarmed civilians or guerrilla forces, without protective equipment, and with little or no capability for destroying the enemy aircraft. The attacks allegedly occurred in remote jungle areas which made confirmation of the attack or recovery of the agent extremely difficult. However, there is enough evidence to suggest that the attacks did indeed take place.

In 1979, a deadly cloud of anthrax was accidentally released from Soviet Military Compound 19, a microbiology facility, in Sverdlovsk, USSR. Although the Soviet Ministry of Health initially cited contaminated meat as the source of the illness, in 1992 Russian President Boris Yeltsin acknowledged the accident involved the escape of anthrax spores from the military research facility and resulted in the death of 66 people who were downwind from Compound 19.

In 1978, a Bulgarian exile named Georgi Markov was murdered by a tiny pellet containing highly poisonous ricin toxin which was fired into his leg by an assassination device disguised as an umbrella. While waiting for a bus on a busy London street, he felt a sharp pain in his calf. He died several days later and the tiny pellet was discovered in his leg upon autopsy. The murder, it was later revealed, was carried out by the communist Bulgarian government with technology supplied by the Soviet Union.

Today, Iraq is at the center of World attention over concern it is developing and stockpiling biological weapons of mass destruction. There are numerous examples of biological and chemical weapons use by the Iraqis during their war with Iran and against their own "undesirable" citizens in times of internal unrest. When United Nations inspectors carried out their inspections after the Gulf War, it became evident that the Iraqis had conducted research and development work on anthrax, botulinum toxins, Clostridium perfringens, aflatoxins, wheat cover smut, and ricin.

Not only had Iraq developed the biological agents, they also had a means of delivery and tested the various delivery systems, including spray tanks, aerial bombs, and rockets. As noted by USAMRIID publications, "In December 1990, the Iraqis filled one hundred R400 bombs with botulinum toxin, fifty with anthrax, and sixteen with aflatoxin. These weapons were deployed in January 1991 to four locations. All in all, Iraq produced 19,000 liters of concentrated botulinum toxin (nearly 10,000 liters filled into munitions), 8,500 liters of concentrated anthrax (6,500 liters filled into munitions) and 2,200 liters of aflatoxin (1,580 liters filled into munitions).

All indications are that the program in Iraq is ongoing, as is evidenced by daily news reports. The current threat is so serious that in December, 1997, the Department of Defense decided to initiate anthrax immunization in U.S. Forces. The operational forces received their first shot of the six shot immunization series in March, 1998.

The problem is getting worse. The January 29, 1998 issue of The *Washington Post* revealed a collaborative effort between Saddam Hussein's Iraq and Moammar Gadhafi's Libya to develop biological weapons. A contingent of Iraqi scientists are conducting a covert research and development program at the Ibn Hayan biological weapons plant in Tripoli, Libya. Libya already has two of the largest chemical weapons production facilities in the developing world, at Rabta and Tarhunah. Given the country's support of terrorist operations, this development is most worrisome.

The Tarhunah facility was built inside a mountain range about 50 miles southeast of Tripoli with the expressed purpose of manufacturing chemical and biological weapons. Covering over six square miles and composed of a labyrinth of tunnels, it was designed to withstand a direct hit from nuclear weapons.

Even extremist groups and terrorists have developed an interest in biological weapons. Members of the Japanese cult, Aum Shinrikyo, responsible for the March 1995 Sarin gas attacks in the Tokyo subway which killed 12 people and injured 5,000 others, reportedly went to Zaire during a recent deadly outbreak of Ebola to obtain samples of the virus.

The use of biological agents as weapons of terror against civilian populations is a growing threat. It has become commonplace to find daily mention of biological weapons in the newspaper or on radio and television.

As a weapon of terror, biological weapons are relatively unique in their ability to cause high numbers of casualties over a large area at minimal expense and by a means which can be virtually untraceable. These weapons are easy to produce, difficult to detect, and hard to protect against. Treating massive numbers of biological casualties would quickly overwhelm the health care systems of even the most advanced countries.

As noted in the latest edition of the NATO handbook, "as the military and economic gaps between nations grow and as some less advantaged nations seek a balance of power, there may be a tendency by these nations to overcome their disadvantage by choosing weapons of mass destruction that can be produced easily and cheaply. The purely financial advantage of employing biological weapons was clearly illustrated by a 1969 expert United Nations panel which estimated the cost of operations against civilian populations at $1 per square kilometer for biological weapons, versus $600 per square kilometer for chemical, $800 per square kilometer nuclear, and $2000 per square kilometer for conventional armaments."

The World Health Organization noted in a 1970 study that fifty kilograms (110 pounds) of aerosolized anthrax spores dispensed 2 kilometers (1.2 miles) upwind of a population center of 500,000 unprotected people in ideal meteorological conditions would travel greater than 20 kilometers (12 miles) downwind and kill up to 220,000 people.

Whether preparing to defend against biological weapons or just combating a naturally occurring infectious disease, comprehensive knowledge of the disease producing organism is vital. Characteristics important to understand include infectivity (a measure of how easy it is to establish an infection), virulence (how severe a disease is produced), toxicity (how severe a disease is produced by a particular toxin), pathogenicity (a reflection of the capability of an infectious agent to cause disease in a susceptible host or target organism), incubation period (the amount of time between exposure to the infective agent and the onset of symptoms), transmissibility (a measure of the ease which infection is passed from person to person), lethality (a measure of the capability of an agent to produce death), and stability (how impervious it is to environmental factors such as sunlight, temperature, and humidity.)

The same types of infectious agents causing natural disease in humans can be modified or "weaponized" to induce disease in an enemy population. Natural disease causing infectious agents include bacteria (anthrax, cholera, plague, shigella, tularemia, typhoid fever), viruses (Ebola, smallpox, yellow fever), Rickettsiae (Q fever, Rocky Mountain spotted fever), Chlamydia (psittacosis), Fungi (coccidioidomycosis, histoplasmosis), and Toxins (botulinum, ricin.)

To be an effective weapon, the biological agent must be dispersed or disseminated to cause disease. This dissemination may involve the same routes of entry as natural disease, i.e. through ingestion, by skin contact, or by inhalation.

Direct contamination of food or water supplies is most suitable for sabotage activities against relatively limited targets. Proper packaging and preparation of food, as well as filtration and adequate chlorination of water will significantly reduce the effectiveness of this threat.

Fortunately, intact skin provides a fairly effective barrier to most biological agents. Mucus membranes and broken skin, however, allow the ready ingress of micro-organisms and toxins.

Since humans require a continual supply of oxygen, and the removal of carbon dioxide, to sustain life, the natural process of breathing provides an avenue by which to expose an individual to a continuing influx of biological agent. The lungs are composed of tiny air sacs, called alveoli, where the exchange of oxygen and carbon dioxide between the air and blood occur. The total surface area of these alveoli in the average adult is about 300 square meters or the size of a tennis court. This large surface area allows for rapid absorption of inhaled materials. Indeed, studies have demonstrated certain drugs instilled into the lungs reach the blood stream as rapidly as they do by direct intravenous injection.

Unfortunately, this is of great advantage to the weapons designer. It makes inhalation the most likely route of attack and allows the dissemination of a biological agent to be accomplished covertly through the use of almost invisible aerosols.

The size of the aerosol droplet is very important, as the major risk of inhaled particles come from those which are retained in the lung tissue. If the particles are too large they will be filtered out in the upper airways by natural bodily defenses and will not reach the lungs. If they are too small they will remain suspended in the inhaled air and will be exhaled. One of the vital questions answered by the CD-22 project was what particle sizes would be of most concern. It was shown that particles between 0.5–5 microns would reach and be retained in the lung air sacs or alveoli.

Other methods of dissemination could include releasing natural reservoirs of infectious agents, i.e. mosquitoes, ticks, or fleas. Person to person spread is also highly effective for some biological agents. The direct person to person spread of the 1918 influenza epidemic is an historical example. The recent Ebola virus epidemics in Africa is a more chillingly modern one.

The ability of the United States to defend it's citizens and armed forces from biological threats follows directly from the pioneering work which was performed during the CD-22 and White-coat projects. Recognition of the importance of this work in preserving the liberty and health of free people around the World will continue to grow.

FORT DETRICK

The story is told of an attempt to create disease by contaminating the drinking water of Chicago during World War I. The attempt was thwarted only as lightning illuminated the dark, stormy night and exposed the figure of the saboteur high on the water tower. Supposedly, the incident was not released to the press in order to avoid mass hysteria. Intelligence also provided reports that during World War II, both Germany and Japan had the capability to employ biological weapons should these be deemed necessary. Thus it was in the fall of 1941, Secretary of War Henry L. Stimson made the following request of the President of the National Academy of Sciences:

Because of the dangers that might confront this nation from potential enemies employing biological warfare, it seems advisable that investigations be initiated to survey the present situation and the future possibilities. I am therefore asking if you will undertake the appointment of an appropriate committee to survey all phases of this matter (Richard M. Clendenin, Science and Technology at Fort Detrick 1943–1968, *U.S. Army, 1968 p. ix).*

The War Bureau of Consultation (WBC) was formed with the mandate to do its work with much secrecy in order not to alert potential enemies of the nation. While biological warfare concepts had been discussed from time to time prior to late 1941, they seemed so far removed as to be deemed impractical.

After careful study, the WBC deemed biological warfare a distinct possibility and proposed that preparations for defense be started immediately. In February 1942 the WBC wrote to Secretary Stimson:

There is but one logical course to pursue, namely, to study the possibilities of such warfare from every angle, make every preparation for reducing its effectiveness, and thereby reduce the likelihood of its use (ibid. p. x).

In May 1942, President Roosevelt authorized Mr. Stimson to create such a sub-unit, the War Research Service (WRS), within the Federal Security Agency. Thus obscured, the WRS became a reality with George W. Merck as director. The WRS was largely civilian operated in order to enhance its research secrecy while avoiding undue alarm in the American populace.

Following the Japanese submarine shelling of a California oil field at Goleta, near Santa Barbara, in December 1941, keen interest in preventing damages by biological warfare increased. Protective measures to prevent contamination of water supplies, milk, food, vaccines and serums were speedily undertaken. The Federal Bureau of Investigation as well as military agencies were utilized to ferret out enemy intentions insofar as biological warfare was concerned. Meanwhile, the WRS organized a research and development program to extend the knowledge of pathogenic agents for offensive use as well as in defense against them

As the program began to fall into place, it became obvious that the problem was too large and too complex for success unless there were some larger scale developmental plans and operations. In November 1942, the WRS requested that the U.S. Army Chemical Warfare Service become responsible for a large-scale research and development operation to include specially-designed laboratories and pilot plants. The site selected was Detrick Field (formerly called Frederick Field), which was a small National Guard Air Field on the outskirts of Frederick, Maryland. Because of the medical hazards inherent in such research, which required close observation of all personnel around the clock, it was deemed best if the research project be totally militarized. The reason for this was that should there be a serious accident befalling civilian employees, security could be better maintained, avoiding possible political complications at home and abroad.

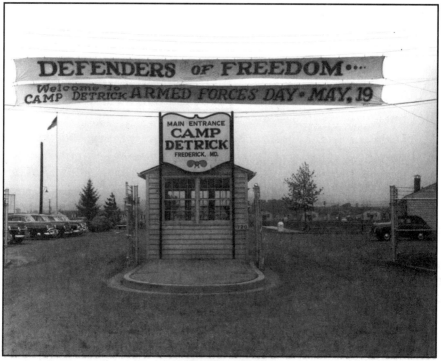

Entering Camp Detrick
US Army Photo

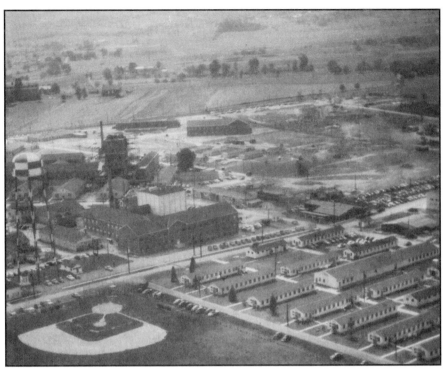

Aerial View (circa late 40's)
US Army Photo

Located in the rolling hills of Maryland, Detrick Field was selected because of its proximity to Washington, D.C. as well as to Edgewood Arsenal, which was (and still is) the Chemical Warfare Service Research Center. An additional reason was that the airplane hanger would be immediately available for housing of research activities while new facilities were being constructed. In addition, there was room for expansion on the 90-acre airfield should this become desirable.

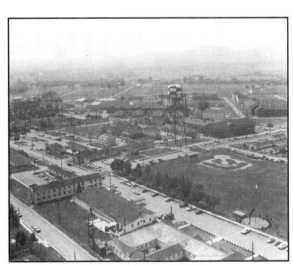

Fort Detrick—Looking West
US Army Photo

Detrick Field had been named in memory of Doctor Frederick L. Detrick, Major, Medical Corps,

Maryland National Guard, and Flight Surgeon of the 104th Observation Squadron, 29th Division, Maryland National Guard, until his death in 1931. Doctor Detrick had served with distinction in France as an Army Medical Officer during World War I. At the time of its purchase by the United States Government, Detrick Field was the home field of Doctor Detrick's squadron and was being utilized for training of student pilots of the Armed

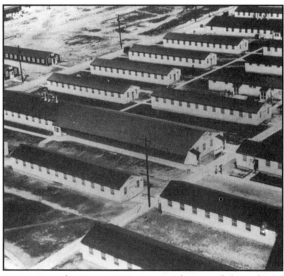

Camp Detrick, Sept. 1944: An aerial view of the enlisted men's barracks. The two long building at left center and upper right was completely renovated in 1961 and served as Headquarters, Fort Detrick, until 1968. It was demolished when the new headquarters building was constructed.

US Army Photo

Forces. When purchased in April 1943, the War Department renamed Detrick Field as Camp Detrick.

Biological, chemical, and mechanical means of protecting the American populace had to be studied. Vaccines, toxoids, antibiotics, disinfectants, and antiseptics had to be carefully evaluated, all the while developing techniques for detecting, sampling, and identifying many pathogens and their toxic products. Simultaneously, sterilization procedures and decontamination protocols required development and improvement. For example, the mask used against gas needed to be a million times more effective in order to effectively filter out biological particles. Activities

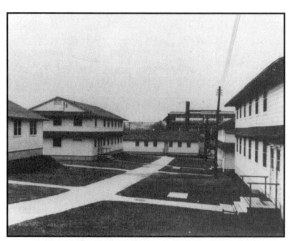

Camp Detrick as it looked in 1943. These buildings were the barracks and mess hall. (US Army Photo)

in Camp Detrick required techniques skills, and concepts not previously fully developed.

By September 1943, the Detrick Safety Division had established, monitored and maintained such tight safety procedures that no biological accidents ever affected the nearby civilian community. In spite of the hazards of experimentation with a variety of highly pathogenic organisms, the magnitude of the operation, and the large number of individuals so involved, during the war years there were only 60 instances of accidental infections that required treatment. Another 159 cases of exposure to pathogens were promptly treated, thus preventing infection. Even these occurrences provided information regarding the efficiency of new antibiotics, immunization procedures, and therapies.

In order to be effective in defense against biological warfare, it was necessary not only to understand medical factors, but also to know how such bacteria could be delivered upon either troop or civilian populace. Medical research in defensive biological warfare thus required a comprehensive knowledge of optimal conditions essential for use of such bacteria as weapons as well as the amounts required. Most Americans had very limited knowledge, or even awareness, of the use of bacteria as a weapon prior to World War II. Growth in public knowledge of health has multiplied perhaps faster than any other single arena in the years since World War II.

Frankly, it is astonishing that medical knowledge and techniques with regard to airborne diseases were so limited in the 1930's and 1940's. For example, what about diseases spread by fleas, ticks, lice, mosquitoes? Could infections, with their causative organisms, be induced through the respiratory system? If so, how, and in what dose size to be effective for each disease? What size would an infectious particle have to be in order to create infections? So, starting with one bacterial toxin and one vegetative organism, research rapidly expanded into a large array of pathogens which might be grown in artificial media. It was deemed necessary to learn about plant diseases and how to cause them or stop them, since such might be used to destroy the nation's food crops, important because history reveals that defeat has more often followed famine and disease than battle losses.

On 3 January 1946, the Department of War issued for the first time a press release informing the American public that Camp Detrick had been involved in research and development of biological warfare. In November 1945, the Military Chiefs of Staff authorized technical research presentations and papers to be publicly released. Since that time, there has been an ongoing flow of such material appearing in scientific journals. This information flow encompasses bacteriology, physiology, pathology, clinical and preventive medicine, veterinary medicine, biochemistry, neurology, mycology, phytopathology, botany, public health, industrial hygiene, instrumentation, chemistry, chemical engineering, and agriculture. From the foregoing areas of research, Operation Whitecoat can be seen as a small part of a rather major research effort.

Early in 1942, research was begun on rinderpest, a disease which kills more than 90 percent of infected animals in areas where it is endemic. Due to the extensive use of meat in the American diet, possible infection by rinderpest in America would be quite serious. Research resulted in a vaccine that may be used to protect native and European cattle against rinderpest. In like manner, research against fowl plague and Newcastle disease, both very serious afflictions of poultry, resulted in an effective vaccine against that disease. It also was demonstrated that hog cholera could be transmitted by airborne aerosols carrying infectious particles of the virus just as aerosols of Newcastle disease could infect healthy chickens.

From the early days of 1941, when the War Bureau of Consultation was created, the Surgeon General of the Army maintained close contact with all aspects of biological warfare research and development, but was not solely in charge of nor totally responsible for the program. In 1956, however, the Army Medical Unit was activated at Fort Detrick with the mission to evaluate the threat of biological warfare and to develop appropriate prophylactic and therapeutic defensive measures, including perfection of both rapid and effective diagnostic and identification procedures. The medical unit was under the Commanding General, Army Medical Research and Development Command, but drew administrative and logistical support from Walter Reed Army Medical Center.

On 3 February 1956 the Department of the Army changed the name of Camp Detrick to Fort Detrick, indicative of a permanent facility. During the passing years, Fort Detrick has become the home of several tenant units and has changed from a small, isolated military camp to a significant research center. It has evolved from an inexpensive airfield into a multi-million dollar research center where medical research on infectious diseases continues for the benefit of mankind. Many of the vaccines developed for diseases studied in the 1950's have been used to save thousands of lives, both in America and abroad. (Incidentally, while Fort Detrick is a U.S. Army post, the U.S. Navy Medical Department has been an active participant in research at that post, having had at one time some 589 personnel, including 134 WAVES on duty by V-E Day in 1945.)

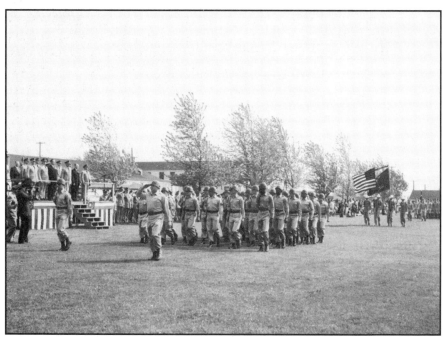

Daily life included drill, ceremonies, parades and military duties as well as the medical work and research. (US Army Photo)

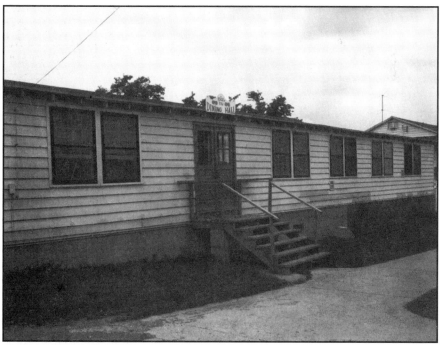

The Dining Hall - Mess Hall - offered welcome relief from hospital food...but not quite like home cooking. (US Army Photo)

For greater details regarding the history of Fort Detrick, see Clendenin, *ibid.* The booklet is available from the Public Information Office at Fort Detrick, Maryland.

OPERATION WHITECOAT

Operation Whitecoat. What was it? Where did it occur? What was its purpose? What were and are the results? Why were Seventh-day Adventists in North America so involved in what was essentially a United States Army medical research project? What were the moral and/or ethical questions posed then, and do such issues continue today? How did the Seventh-day Adventist Church become involved in this issue? Such questions were raised at the inception of Operation Whitecoat, and echoes of these questions still reverberate from time to time.

The genesis of such concepts, leading to the development of Operation Whitecoat, began during World War II as a result of concerns raised by biological and chemical endeavors of the German and Japanese militaries. Operation Whitecoat (also called Project Whitecoat) is an outgrowth of military research that began as defensive measures should chemical or biological warfare be instituted against the United States. Initially under the joint control of the U.S. Army Chemical Corps and the U.S. Army Medical Service, the research had been divided by 1954 into the Army Chemical Command and the Army Medical Department, functioning as the Army Medical Research Unit, with the latter being situated at the Army's Walter Reed Hospital in Washington, DC. The Army Medical Research Unit was later named the United States Army Medical Research Institute of Infectious Diseases. In typical military style, it has become known as USAMRIID (pronounced "you-sam-rid"). Operation Whitecoat was but one component of a much larger military medical research endeavor.

As its name implies, USAMRIID does research in infectious diseases, with a focus of defense against possible natural or enemy use of infectious agents. All the diseases researched to date and reported in scientific accounts are frequently found naturally occurring in many areas of the world, including the United States. Medical records reveal that more military personnel are incapacitated or die due to disease than by violent enemy action. Self preservation requires serious attention to those preventative procedures that promote health for both the military and civilian communities. Operation Whitecoat, like its predecessors, was to develop defenses against naturally-acquired diseases as well as against microorganisms that might be used against the military or the civilian communities. Much of Operation Whitecoat medical research in defensive biological warfare focused on possibilities, methodologies and defenses of airborne infections.

USAMRIID is physically located at Fort Detrick, Frederick, Maryland, about fifty miles northwest of Washington, D.C. The decision to place the Army Medical Research Unit there was based on several factors that included proximity to the U.S. Army Walter Reed Medical

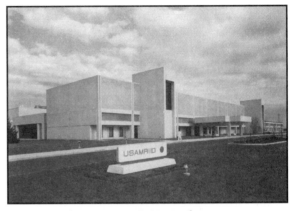

The new USAMRIID Headquarters

US Army Photo

Center; the research facilities already located there; and the interfacing of personnel of the Medical Center and the Research Unit. The Walter Reed Medical Center is perhaps the pre-eminent or most prestigious U.S. Army hospital in the world, just as the U.S. Naval Hospital at Bethesda, Maryland, and the U.S. Air Force Wilfred Hall Hospital in San Antonio, Texas, are for the Navy and Air Force.

Inasmuch as USAMRIID is located at Fort Detrick, Maryland, which is also the historic Research Center for Chemical Warfare, some individuals quickly assumed that USAMRIID was also engaged in researching infectious diseases for offensive purposes rather than as defense should this type of warfare be used against America and/or its Allies. Because responsible scientific research findings are normally reported at professional meetings and in technical scientific journals, versus the popular press or news media, some individuals were convinced that USAMRIID's Operation Whitecoat was engaged in dark, deep, sinister research. With such beliefs, it was quite natural for some individuals to become critical.

Intensive medical research and experimentation for such illnesses as Q fever, tularemia, Eastern, Western and Venezuelan equine encephalomyelitis, and sandfly fever, typhoid fever, Rocky Mountain fever, spotted tick fever, Rift Valley fever, and others, were executed. Additionally, Operation Whitecoat tested and compared gas masks, isolation suits (which were eventually utilized for space exploration), the effects of sleep deprivation, et cetera.

Why was the Seventh-day Adventist Church was so closely identified and involved in Operation Whitecoat? To adequately answer this question requires an awareness of the historic development of the Church theologically and organizationally.

With its strong emphasis upon health and medical care, perhaps no other church of comparable size has so many hospitals, clinics, and health food factories world wide. The espoused philosophy of biblically-based health concepts and practices, combined with the teachings of responsible citizenship, emphasis on the Great Commission of the Gospel to all the world, and the Church's encouragement of its youthful adherents to seriously consider noncombatancy, led many drafted Seventh-day Adventists to volunteer for Operation Whitecoat when the opportunity was presented. A large number of these young Adventist military draftees seem to have strongly believed that participation in medical research might well benefit both their fellow servicemen and the civilian community at large.

It would be naive, however, to think that all such volunteers did so solely for altruistic reasons, even though nothing would be illegal, immoral, or unethical if other factors were also involved. Most of life's decisions are made for multiple reasons and seldom for just one. Why should the decision of how to spend two years of enforced military service be any different?

The story of Operation Whitecoat needs to be told not only to illuminate the effort and sacrifice of those who volunteered, but to examine and carefully evaluate it's moral and bioethical implications.

Operation Whitecoat was unique in the annals of American history as it was the first time the United States military sought cooperation from a particular church organization to form its cadre of volunteers. From a research perspective, there were valid reasons for this approach. There also appears to have been some logical reasons for the General Conference of Seventh-day Adventists to view the objectives of Operation Whitecoat with favor.

To fully understand and appreciate why the Army Medical Department and the Seventh-day Adventist Church in North America cooperated in Operation Whitecoat, it is imperative that one study the attitudes and relationships of the Seventh-day Adventist Church to the military since the Church's inception in the first half of the nineteenth century.

An awareness of the cooperative relationship between the military and the Church in medical and health activities during times of war is also helpful. For instance, during World War II the Army's 47th General Hospital in the Pacific Theatre was staffed primarily by Adventist personnel from White Memorial Hospital and from Loma Linda University Medical School (then called College of Medical Evangelists) and Medical Center, both institutions being "flag ships" in the worldwide Adventist hospital system. These individuals, as well as the thousands of other Adventist medical, dental, and nursing officers and enlisted personnel, were prime examples of health care concerns in the fight against disease. The Adventist Church's sense of the "Great Commission" has caused it to be deeply involved in health care around the world. Thus the concept of Operation Whitecoat was seen to be harmonious with the Church's long-established medical and health care concepts and practices.

While hundreds of research projects in infectious diseases have taken place and are ongoing, this volume limits itself to Operation Whitecoat. Although numerous studies have been presented in professional meetings and in scientific journals, there does not seem to be any single report providing an overall perspective of Operation Whitecoat. The experiences and emotions of most Operation Whitecoat volunteers have not been related. This is essential if the full story is to be known. In an attempt to accomplish this, a serious and sustained effort was made to contact all Operation Whitecoat volunteers, as well as those major figures of USAMRIID involved in Operation Whitecoat over the years of its existence.

In late 1976, Brigadier General William S. Augerson, Medical Corps., U.S. Army Commanding Surgeon General, Research and Development Program, wrote a letter to someone who had inquired about Operation Whitecoat. The relevant portion of his letter is quoted here, as it gives an excellent overview of the project. (The original letter is in the General Conference Archives, Project Whitecoat files.)

Project White coat is the designation used to identify the human volunteer program associated with medical research conducted by the US. Army Medical Research Institute of Infectious Diseases at Fort Detrick, Maryland (prior to January 1969 designated The US Army Medical Unit). This volunteer program originated in 1955 following a series of meetings between representatives of the General Conference of the Seventh-day Adventist Church and the Office of the Surgeon General of the Army.

The purpose of Project White coat was to utilize human volunteers in medical studies to evaluate the effect of certain biological pathogens upon humans in an effort to determine the vulnerability of man to attack with biological agents. Additionally, the studies were conducted and designed to develop and improve the United States' medical defense against biological warfare by developing more rapid means of medical identification of biological agents, improving methods of treatment and prophylaxis and developing vaccines for immunization for protection of all United States' forces who might be subjected to offensive biological warfare or sent to parts of the world where certain infectious diseases are endemic in nature.

When the program was initially implemented in 1955, it was under the command and control of the Walter Reed Army Institute of Research (WRAIR). On 20 June 1956, by General Order No. 37, Headquarters, Walter Reed Army Medical Center, the U.S. Army Medical Unit (USAMU) was established at Fort Detrick, Maryland and the Project Whitecoat program came under command and control of the USA MU. General Order No 9, Office of the Surgeon General, dated 29 September 1958, assigned the USAMU to Headquarters, U.S. Army Medical Research and Development Command. General Order No. 6, Office of the Surgeon General, dated 27 January 1969, redesignated The USAMU as the U.S. Army Medical Research Institute of Infectious Diseases (USAMRIID), which is the current designation.

Personnel for Project Whitecoat were recruited from military personnel with a 1-A-O (conscientious objector) classification who were undergoing Basic and Advanced Individual Training at the U.S. Army Medical Center at Fort Sam Houston, Texas. Twice a year, the Commander and Executive Training of the Medical Unit, and the Director of the National Service Organization of the Seventh-day Adventist General Conference, interviewed personnel at the Medical Training Center to select personnel for Project Whitecoat. These personnel were given an explanation of the program to include discussion of the risks involved. Personnel were offered an opportunity to ask questions about the program.

All participation was voluntary and with the knowing consent of the individual. He was able to exercise free power of choice without undue inducement. Based on the interviews and the research needs of the Medical Unit, a number of these personnel, who were medically qualified, were selected and assigned to the Medical Unit upon completion of their training at Fort Sam Houston, Texas.

Upon arrival at the Medical Unit, each Project Whitecoat volunteer underwent a thorough medical examination which included a complete medical history, a detailed physical examination and extensive laboratory studies. Upon completion of the physical examination and administrative processing, each volunteer was then assigned to such duties as medical maintenance technician, animal caretaker, etc. Volunteers in the program were assigned these duties as only about twenty percent of their duty time was spent actually engaged in research studies. Each individual volunteer was considered a full time soldier and received no special consideration for participating in medical research studies.

Prior to any medical research study being conducted, Project Whitecoat personnel were called together, given a comprehensive briefing as to the purpose and nature of the study, the risk involved and exactly what was expected of each participant. After any questions that might arise had been answered for the group, each subject was interviewed and then asked to indicate his desire regarding participation in the study. If the individual desired to participate in the study, he then was required to sign a consent form. Any individual who did not desire to participate in the study was not required to do so. Prior to the actual study beginning, every volunteer was again given a thorough medical evaluation to assure that they were medically fit to participate in the study.

Adequate facilities were provided and proper study conditions were stringently addressed to protect the human subject against all foreseeable possibilities of injury or disability. The highest degree of skill and care was required during all stages of the study of persons conducting or assisting in the study.

The use of Seventh-day Adventists in Project White coat terminated in 1973. This was brought about by the elimination of the draft which was the mechanism for bringing conscientious objectors into the service. From the beginning of Project Whitecoat in 1955 until 1973, some 2,200 Seventh-day Adventists participated in this program. Their unselfish and humane contributions have helped to advance medical science and enabled military medical researchers to progress in their knowledge of infectious diseases and their development of methods for treatment, prophylaxis and immunization.

THE GENESIS

In order to continue and to expand the Army's research in infectious diseases and vaccines using human volunteers, the proposed project was examined exceedingly carefully with regard to legal, ethical and moral issues. Attention to these issues resulted in operating requirements and procedures precluding the disregard for the health or life of any volunteer. The program operated for almost 20 years without a single fatality among those who participated in Operation Whitecoat.

Almost two years prior to the authorization of Operation Whitecoat, an ad hoc committee had been formed by the Army Medical Corps to investigate biological warfare defense by inoculating volunteers with Coxiella burnetii, the infectious agent causing Q fever. This served as the prototypical biologic warfare agent, and by studying the effects of curable infectious disease, one can develop treatments and protective measures against the incurable.

This project was known as the CD-22 program. The focus of CD-22 project was study of the vulnerability of the human being to biological agents, the prevention of and treatment of biological warfare casualties, the identification of biological agents, determination of minimum effective dosages, the effectiveness of prophylactic and therapeutic measures, the serologic responses to infections, and the effects of various doses of inoculum. CD-22 research efforts were terminated in 1956 after yielding the first scientific data of its kind and providing answers to most of the questions which had led to the study. The entire CD-22 program was monitored by the Commission on Epidemiological Survey of the Armed Forces Epidemiological Board. Thereafter, responsibility to provide defenses against biological warfare was assigned to the Army medical services under the purview of the Surgeon General. Medical research would continue, but totally within the medical structure of the military. A precedent had been established, as CD-22 pioneered scientific medical research using volunteer human subjects.

The successes of the CD-22 project, the development of legal guidelines, and the delineation of responsibilities concerning defensive medical biological warfare research led to the establishment of the United States Army Medical Unit (USAMU) on 20 June 1956, with personnel from both Walter Reed Army Hospital and Camp Detrick. Part of USAMU's responsibility was to research and develop a defense against biological warfare. Colonel W. D. Tigertt, Medical Corps, United States Army, assumed command of USAMU and continued in command until 1961. As commander, Colonel Tigertt developed a close rapport with the Seventh-day Adventist

Church so that the flow of Adventist volunteers to Operation White-coat continued after his departure, and lasted until the Selective Service draft ended in 1972.

Having carried the research of particular infectious diseases and potential vaccines as far as possible on animals, the Army medical researchers believed it was now time for human trials. The Army Medical Department wanted its' research to conform to the highest ethical standards, unlike research some previously conducted on humans.

Historical documents clearly demonstrate that medical research and experimentation on humans became institutionalized on a large scale during World War II by both parties of that conflict. Disease was perceived to be the enemy, and both sides desperately wanted cures for diseases that were crippling their military efforts.

Illnesses such as dysentery, malaria, and venereal diseases seemed more effective than bombs or bullets. While such experiments were fully supported by governmental funding, these were not the first large-scale research projects to use human beings as research objects. Lest we fault the military, similar research was also carried on in the civilian community. Doctor Devoid J. Rothman, in an article titled "Ethics and Human Experimentation: Henry Beecher Revisited" *(The New England Journal of Medicine,* vol. 317:19 pp. 1194–219) states:

The wartime environment also undercut the protection of human subjects, because of the power of the example of the draft. Every day thousands of men were compelled to risk death, however limited their understanding of the aims of the war. By extension, researchers doing laboratory work were also engaged in a military activity, and they did not feel the need to seek the permission of their subjects anymore than the selective service or field commanders did of draftees. In a society mobilized for war, these arguments carried great weight. Some people were ordered to face bullets and storm a hill; others were told to take an injection and test a vaccine. In philosophical terms wartime inevitability promoted utilitarian over absolutistic positions.

It was only after the war that it became apparent that some researchers had gone far beyond acceptable ethical standards. Historical records show that a number of German physicians, under Nazism, participated in euthanasia programs in which the comatose, the insane, and the gypsies were experimented upon and then deliberately killed. The absence of an outcry against these programs led to the Holocaust. Anopheles mosquitoes were brought in from swamps to transmit malaria to humans for study; particles of glass and stone were introduced into wounds to test the efficacy of new sulfa drugs; Jewish and Russian inmates were stripped and chilled in icy waters or blizzards in order to better understand hypothermia and improve methods of treating German soldiers and airman exposed to cold environments.

In some experiments physicians would shoot captive inmates to study gunshot wounds; some would implant hormones to see if homosexuality could be cured; or starve inmates to study the physiology of nutrition; or surgically remove the legs and arms of women to study regeneration; or as Doctor Mengele did, study the effects of radiation by subjecting a group of Polish nuns to exceedingly high doses.

The Japanese biological warfare laboratory in Harbin, Manchuria has already been discussed and serves as an example that the German experience was not an isolated case.

Human experimentation has a lengthy history, as does the effort to adequately define appropriate guidelines for it. Edward Jenner tested his initial smallpox vaccines on his firstborn son and on neighborhood children. Louis Pasteur worried about the use of humans in testing rabies antidotes. It was only after medical colleagues convinced him that death was inevitable that he used his serum on the child Joseph Meister. German physicians tested a serum against diphtheria on 30 hospitalized patients as a therapeutic procedure. Banting and Best tested insulin therapy on diabetics who were in coma or on its edge. In like manner, the causative agent of syphilis was tested in New York on some 400 subjects, many of whom were mental hospital inmates or orphans in asylums.

The reaction to the attrocities of World War II helped facilitate the development of more closely controlled and humane medical testing. The public outcry when such events were revealed created the climate in which *voluntary* participation, no matter how dangerous it might seem, became the ideal for individual participation in serious medical research. This change was a process rather than a sudden happening. Even so, the transformation occurred within a matter of very few years.

In 1944, the Nuremberg Code was developed as a template for ethical human experimentation and contains the basic elements of voluntary consent, which is still in use today. It reads as follows:

The Nuremberg Code

1. The voluntary consent of the human subject is absolutely essential. This means that the person involved should have legal capacity to give consent; should be situated as to be able to ex-

ercise free power of choice, without the intervention of any element of force, fraud, deceit, duress, overreaching, or other ulterior form of constraint or coercion; and should have sufficient knowledge and comprehension of the elements of the subject matter involved as to enable him to make an understanding and enlightened decision. The latter element requires that before the acceptance of an affirmative decision by the experimental subject there should be made known to him the nature, duration, and purpose of the experiment; the method and means by which it is to be conducted; all inconveniences and hazards reasonably to be expected; and the effects upon his health or person which may possibly come from his participation in the experiments. The duty and responsibility for ascertaining the quality of the consent rest upon each individual who initiates, directs or engages in the experiment. It is a personal duty and responsibility which may not be delegated to another with impunity.

2. The experiment should be such as to yield fruitful results for the good of society, unprocurable by other methods or means of study, and not random and unnecessary in nature.

3. The experiment should be so designed and based on the results of animal experimentation and a knowledge of the natural history of the disease or other problem under study that the anticipated results will justify the performance of the experiment.

4. The experiment should be so conducted as to avoid all unnecessary physical and mental suffering and injury.

5. No experiment should be conducted where there is an a priori reason to believe that death or disabling injury will occur; except, perhaps, in those experiments where the experimental physicians also serve as subjects.

6. The degree of risk to be taken should never exceed that determined by the humanitarian importance of the problem to be solved by the experiment.

7. Proper preparation should be made and adequate facilities provided to protect the experimental subject against even remote possibilities of injury, disability, or death.

8. The experiment should be conducted only by scientifically qualified persons. The highest degree of skill and care should be required through all stages of the experiment of those who conduct or engage in the experiment.

9. During the course of the experiment the human subject should be at liberty to bring the experiment to an end if he has reached the physical or mental state where continuation of the experiment seems to him to be impossible.

10. During the course of the experiment the scientist in charge must be prepared to terminate the experiment at any stage, if he has probable cause to believe, in the exercise of the good faith, superior skill, and care judgment required of him, that a continuation of the experiment is likely to result in injury, disability, or death to the experimental subject.

In order to insure implimentation of these concepts within the Armed Forces, Secretary of Defense Wilson drafted and sent the following memorandum, which was to become known as the Wilson Memorandum, to the chiefs of all the branches of the military services:

SECRETARY OF DEFENSE
Washington

26 FEB 1953

Memorandum for the   SECRETARY OF THE ARMY
                                SECRETARY OF THE NAVY
                                SECRETARY OF THE AIR FORCE

SUBJECT: Use of Human Volunteers in Experimental Research

1. Based upon a recommendation of the Armed Forces Medical Policy Council, that human subjects be employed, under recognized safeguards, as the only feasible means for realistic evaluation and/or development of effective preventive measures of defense against atomic, biological or chemical agents, the policy set forth below will govern the use of human volunteers by the Department of Defense in esperimental research in the fields of atomic, biological and/or chemical warfare.

2. By reason of the basic medical responsibility in connection with the development of defense of all types against atomic, biological and/or chemical warfare agents, Armed Services personnel and/or civilians on duty at installations engaged in such research shall be permitted to actively participate in all phases of the program, such participation shall be subject to the following conditions:

a. The voluntary consent of the human subject is absolutely essential.

1. This means that the person involved should have legal capacity to give consent; should be so situated as to be able to exercise free power of choice, without the intervention of any element of force, fraud, deceit, duress, overreaching, or other ulterior form of constraint or coercion; and should have sufficient knowledge and comprehension of the elements of the subject matter involved as to enable him to make an understanding and enlightened decision. This latter element requires that before the acceptance of an affirmative decision by the experimental subject there should be made known to him the nature, duration, and purpose of the experiment; the method and means by which it is to be conducted; all inconveniences and hazards reasonably to be expected; and the effects upon his health or person which may possibly come from his participation in the experiment.

2. The concept [sic: consent] of the human subject shall be in writing, his signature shall be affixed to a written instrument setting forth substantially the aforementioned requirements and shall be signed in the presence of at least one witness who shall attest to such signature in writing.

a. In experiments where personnel from more than one Service are involved the Secretary of the Service which is exercising primary responsibility for conducting the experiment is designated to prepare such an instrument and coordinate it for use by all the Services having human volunteers involved in the experiment.

3. The duty and responsibility for ascertaining the quality of the consent rests upon each individual who initiates, directs or engages in the experiment. It is a personal duty and responsibility which may not be delegated to another with impunity.

b. The experiment should be such as to yield fruitful results for the good of society, unprocurable by other methods or means of study, and not random and unnecessary in nature.

c. The number of volunteers used shall be kept at a minimum consistent with item b., above.

d. The experiment should be so designed and based on the results of animal experimentation and a knowledge of the natural history of the disease or other problem under study that the anticipated results will justify the performance of the experiment.

e. The experiment should be so conducted as to avoid all unnecessary physical and mental suffering and injury.

f. No experiment should be so conducted where there is an a priori reason to believe that death or disabling injury will occur.

g. The degree of risk to be taken should never exceed that determined by the humanitarian importance of the problem to be solved by the experiment.

h. Proper preparation should be made and adequate facilities provided to protect the experimental subject against even remote possibilities of injury, disability, or death.

i. The experiment should be conducted only by scientifically qualified persons. The highest degree of skill and care should be required through all stages of the experiment of those who conduct or engage in the experiment.

j. During the course of the experiment, the human subject should be at liberty to bring the experiment to an end if he has reached the physical or mental state where continuation of the experiment seems to him to be impossible.

k. During the course of the experiment, the scientist in charge must be prepared to terminate the experiment at any stage if he has probable cause to believe, in the exercise of the good faith, superior skill and careful judgment required of him, that a continuation of the experiment is likely to result in injury, disability or death to the experimental subject.

l. The established policy, which prohibits the use of prisoners of war in human experimentation, is continued and they will not be used under any circumstances.

3. The Secretaries of the Army, Navy, and Air Force are authorized to conduct experiments in connection with the development of defenses of all types against atomic, biological and/or chemical warfare agents involving the use of human subjects within the limits prescribed above.

4. In each instance in which an experiment is proposed pursuant to this memorandum, the nature and purpose of the proposed experiment and the name of the person who will be in charge of such experiment shall be submitted for approval to the Secretary of the military department in which the proposed experiment is to be conducted. No such experiment shall be undertaken until such Secretary has approved in writing the experiment proposed, the person who will be in charge of conducting it, as well as informing the Secretary of Defense.

5. The addresses [sic] will be responsible for insuring compliance with the provisions of this memorandum within their respective Services.

/signed/
C.E. WILSON

Copies furnished:
 Joint Chiefs of Staff
 Research and Development Board

TOP SECRET Downgraded to UNCLASSIFIED 22 AUG 75

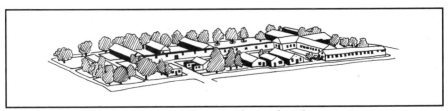

Fort Detrick Hospital Complex during the Whitecoat era.

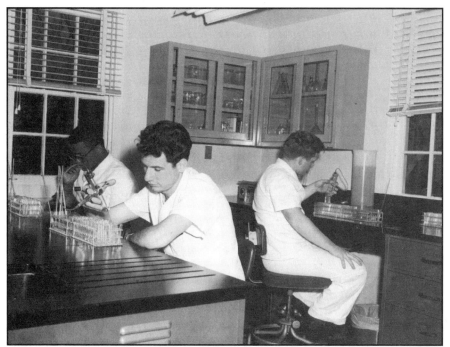

Whitecoat members Howard Wein (center) and Ed Fletcher (right) with Chemical Corps Bill Linthicum in a typical laboratory. (US Army Photo)

Thus it was that on 14 October 1954, Lieutenant Colonel W.D. Tigertt wrote to Major General George F. Armstrong, Medical Corps, Surgeon General, Department of the Army the following letter (General Conference Archives Project Whitecoat):

Several days ago, I contacted Dr. Theodore R. Flaiz, Secretary, Medical Department, General Conference of Seventh-Day [sic] Adventists, to ascertain the views of his church organization as they related to the use of volunteers in medical research.

After I had explained in general terms the type of study which was contemplated, Dr. Flaiz proposed that it should be considered by a small group of the Conference officers and agreed to bring such a group together during the week of 18 October. Dr. Flaiz appeared to be extremely interested and considered it was a real opportunity for members of the Seventh-Day Adventist group to assist in the national defense. It is possible that the church will actively support the project and assist in obtaining the necessary volunteers.

If you consider the attached letter to be appropriate, we believe that it would strengthen our approach to this group materially. I would like to deliver it to Dr. Flaiz at the time of the conference.

This letter to the Surgeon General followed earlier dialogue between Lieutenant Colonel Tigertt and Doctor Flaiz, who was the senior executive of the General Conference Health Department, which had oversight of the world wide health work of the Church. T. R. Flaiz, M.D. had wide experience due to his foreign service in what is now known as Third World countries.

Following the conference with Lieutenant Colonel Tigertt, Doctor Flaiz brought the issue of Adventist participation to the General Conference officers for guidance and instruction. Then at the Officers Meeting on 14 October 1954 (General Conference Archives, *ibid.*), Doctor Flaiz met with them and explained in greater detail the confidential medical research project of the Army. The project would require volunteers to serve as subjects in research experimentation. The minutes of that meeting show that a subcommittee was set up to study the proposal:

Agreed to ask A. V. Olson, T. R. Flaiz, D. E. Rebock, and E. W. Dunbar to study the project with the Army Officer concerned with a view to determining whether or not Seventh-day Adventists could conscientiously participate in the project.

On 18 October 1954, Surgeon General Armstrong responded to Lieutenant Colonel Tigertt's letter with one addressed to Doctor Flaiz (General Conference Archives, *ibid.*):

I have been advised by Lieutenant Colonel W. D. Tigertt, MC, that you have arranged for him to present to representatives of the Seventh-day Adventist Conference a request for their assistance in the conduct of a study of the highest importance to our nation's health. Only through the use of volunteers can the necessary information be obtained.

Colonel Tigertt will explain to you in considerable detail the reasons for and the aims of the program. I want to emphasize, however, that we have sought and received the advice of the leading physicians of the United States in reaching this decision. We have their assurance that they will continue to advise us and, indeed, will directly assist us in this project. The program has the full concurrence of our highest military and governmental officers.

It is my earnest hope that your conference will consider that participation of your men in this program is appropriate. You can thereby make yet another significant contribution to our Nation's health and to our national security.

If during your deliberations questions arise that you feel should be directed to me, I will be glad to meet with you.

With highest personal regards.

On 19 October 1954, Doctor Flaiz responded to the Surgeon General's letter of the previous day in the following way (General Conference Archives, *ibid.*):

Through the courtesy of Colonel W. D. Tigertt, MD, I have just received your letter of October 18.

We have appreciated very much Colonel Tigertt's clear and patient delineation of the plan for the medical research project which you have under way. We feel that if any one should recognize a debt of loyalty and service for the many courtesies and considerations received from the Department of Defense, we, as Adventists, are in a position to feel a debt of gratitude for these kind considerations.

The type of voluntary service which is being offered to our boys in this research program offers an excellent opportunity for these young men to render a service which will be of value not only to military medicine but to public health generally. I believe I speak not only the sentiments of our administrative group in this office, but also of our Adventist young men in the services in observing that it should be regarded as a privilege to be identified with this significant advanced step in clinical research.

As we have indicated to Colonel Tigertt, we will try to have an appropriate statement of our attitude toward this matter in your hands within a few days.

Doctor Flaiz, on 27 October 1954, followed through with another letter to Lieutenant Colonel Tigertt, and enclosed a statement written by the Secretary of the General Conference, W. R. Beach (General Conference Archives, *ibid.*). This statement was sent after its approval by the above-mentioned subcommittee, which voted to support the project as proposed and explained by Lieutenant Colonel Tigertt.

I am sorry to be somewhat delayed in getting into your hands the statement which I promised the other day. We have been very hard pressed with the various meetings of the annual business council of the denomination. We have found time, however, to give study to the matter which you represented to us at the time of your visit, and we feel that the statement accompanying this letter sets forth our attitude toward the type of research work which you have represented to us.

We wish to assure you, Colonel Tigertt, that we as citizens and our young men as soldiers in our national defense forces, wish to do our part in serving the interest of our country.

I would be interested, Colonel Tigertt, in learning something of the results of this research project when it comes through to a successful conclusion.

Wishing you every success in the good work you are doing to advance the cause of health and the welfare of our country.

STATEMENT OF ATTITUDE
REGARDING VOLUNTEERING FOR MEDICAL RESEARCH

Seventh-day Adventists are well aware of the exploits of Pasteur, Gorgas, Reed and their associates by which many of the dangerous and epidemic diseases have been robbed of their terror. Progress in the knowledge of these diseases and in the development of techniques for their control was often achieved through deliberate risk to themselves personally. It is through the risks and dangers which they accepted in line with and beyond the call of duty that we are now comparatively safe from plagues which a generation or two ago claimed their victims in large numbers. We honor these men for their courage and sacrificial devotion to the betterment of the lot of their fellow men.

There are still conspicuous blank spaces in our knowledge of disease and it's treatment. Research in these areas calls for some of the same selfless devotion in the search for lifesaving knowledge as was manifest by the pioneers of modern medicine.

It is the attitude of Seventh-day Adventists that any service rendered voluntarily by whomsoever in the useful necessary research into the cause and the treatment of disabling disease is a legitimate and laudable contribution to the success of our nation and to the health and comfort of our fellow men.

So far as Seventh-day Adventist personnel is concerned, we would earnestly request that the conscientious principles by which our young men live might be respected and guaranteed by the Armed Services in the project the same as it is now in their regular line of military duty.

Following extensive legal review and building on the groundwork already established by Lieutenant Colonel Tigertt, and upon the recommendations of Major Generals W.M. Creasy Chief Chemical Officer, and G.E. Armstrong, Surgeon General of the Army, the Secretary of the Army granted authority to utilize human volunteers in research investigations for defense against biological warfare on 14 January 1955. Then on 21 February 1956, Major Generals Armstrong and Creasy signed a revised agreement, "Responsibilities for the Conduct of Research and Development for Defense Against Biological Warfare" (General Conference Archives, *ibid.)* This document, in conjunction with the Secretary of the Army's policies, governed the research responsibilities of the Army Medical Unit until 1962, when revised agreements were signed.

The Secretary of the Army's authorization of 14 January 1955 provided a new and added dimension to biological warfare research then being conducted. It permitted effective research in development of defenses against the use of microbiological agents which could be scientifically conducted and evaluated without relying upon data extrapolated from animal research. Moreover, it established a standard of human participation that had been grossly ignored heretofore by many researchers.

The proposed and accepted Operation Whitecoat goals and procedures permitted some 2,200 Adventist soldiers to take part in the ongoing medical research at USAMRIID, with an additional 800 men functioning as laboratory technicians, ward attendants, and in other significant roles essential to the project

On 14 September, 1955, the new Surgeon General, U.S. Army Major General C. B. Hayes, wrote the following letter to A. V. Olson, who was Vice President of the General Conference and Chairman of the War Service Commission (General Conference Archives, *op. cit.*):

This letter concerns a number of Adventist young men who have participated voluntarily in a military medical research program and who, by their acts, have contributed materially to the development of knowledge essential to the defense of the United States and to the advancement of medical science. Only through the use of such volunteers could the necessary information have been obtained.

The results obtained become even more meaningful when it is appreciated that the program's inception can be dated from a letter written by my predecessor General Armstrong, to Dr. Flaiz, Secretary of your Medical Department, on October 18, 1954. That many of our aims have been accomplished in this short period of time indicates the nature of the support given by the General Conference, through its War Service Commission, and of the wholehearted participation evinced by your men in uniform.

The reason for this program and the expectations we had for it were described by General Armstrong in his presentation, titled "The Role of the Army Medical Service in the Maintenance of National Health," to the Association of Military Surgeons of the United States, at Washington, DC on November 29, 1954. I would like to quote pertinent parts of this article.

"The Army Medical Service, with its requirement for operation anywhere in the world, must maintain a continuing interest in all of

the communicable diseases. Obviously, should such diseases ever again become problems in this country, the information deriving from these studies would be directly applicable to the overall national health. Our work in these fields is well known and we plan to continue and expand these programs.

"Much of the needed information can be obtained only through the use of volunteers. This fact has been emphasized in resolutions transmitted to the Secretary of Defense by the Division of Medical Sciences of the National Research Council and the American College of Surgeons. Approximately two years ago the Medical Policy Council of the Department of Defense endorsed these statements. It is with considerable pride that I bring to your attention the fact we have never failed to have the fullest cooperation of these self-sacrificing groups of individuals. Our military medical debt to such volunteers, which began with the work on yellow fever has increased markedly in recent years and will continue to grow larger.

"Quantitative data deriving from investigations now in progress is expected to materially enhance our ability to evaluate the magnitude of risk from various specific disease agents from the standpoint of their deliberate introduction into this country by an enemy. Likewise, we expect to obtain a more finite evaluation of our vaccination and chemo-therapy as methods of prophylaxis, to evaluate the role of living agents as vaccines, and to determine the level of effectiveness of our current methods of treatment."

While it will be some months yet before all the medical data can be evaluated, it is completely clear now that, in the Q fever project, in which your group has participated, most of the objectives noted above have been met. For the benefit of non-medical readers I perhaps should explain, as has been explained in detail to each of the volunteers, that Q fever is not a code designation, but the accepted medical name of a disease having a world-wide distribution, and one which was the cause of considerable difficulty to us in World War II. It also occurs in our own country, particularly in the Western States.

It is our belief that each volunteer in this program has been fully aware of the potential hazards of the disease to which he was exposed and we know that in each instance their participation was without promise of reward or material gain. The courage shown by these men is of particular note and, while this letter to you is a form of recognition of the contribution of the group, there will also be recognition of each participant in accordance with military practices.

Although we have had the active support of several members of the General Conference, I would like to make particular mention of the time and energy devoted to this program by the General Secretary of the War Service Commission, Elder G. W. Chambers. In this, as in our numerous other contacts with him, he has shown a broad apprecia- tion of the aims of the Medical Service and of the other participating agencies. He has made himself constantly available, serving as a spiritual leader and as an administrator.

You have my permission to make such public use of this letter as you may deem appropriate. I would hope that if reference to it is made in your denominational publications, you see fit to publish also your own "Statement of Attitude Regarding Volunteering for Medical Re- search." This latter document, to me, constitutes one of the finest gen- eral statements on this important and vital subject that it has ever been my good fortune to read.

The General Conference, as well as the Surgeon General, re- garded the services being rendered by the Adventist Whitecoat vol- unteers so highly that a commendatory article was published in the official church paper, *The Review and Herald* (November 3, 1955. pp. 20–21). This article openly endorsed the Whitecoat program by both the Army and the Church. While colorfully describing the con- tributions of each Whitecoat member, it did so with particular refer- ence to their service for their country and countrymen as well as the individual fortitude demonstrated. This article as much as any sin- gle event influenced the North American Adventist membership and encouraged Army conscientious objectors to volunteer to be a part of USAMRIID's Operation Whitecoat. Both the Army and the Church perceived Whitecoat volunteers to be an extremely valuable if not irreplaceable resource that extended itself beyond the call of duty.

On the occasion of volunteer recruiting visits, the representa- tive of the National Service Organization of the General Conference also made a presentation, for a two-fold purpose. The first was to in- form the potential volunteers of the Church's position and to insure that no misunderstanding would encourage or hinder freedom of choice. The second reason was to assure all that the Church would support each individual's choice, whatever that choice might be. The following is a prototype presentation authored by Clark Smith (General Conference Archives, *op. Cit.*).

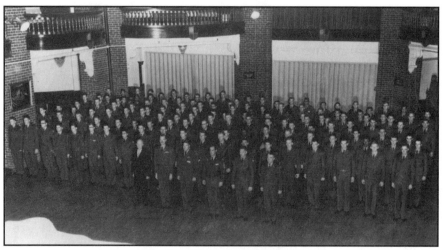

One of the first Whitecoat groups (ca 54–56)

PROJECT WHITECOAT

(A statement by the Director of the National Service Organiza-tion of the General Conference of Seventh-day Adventists to be given to those who are being considered for Project Whitecoat.)

There here are numerous questions that Seventh-day Adventists in the military service commonly ask their church officials about Pro-ject Whitecoat when there is a possibility that they may be given an op-portunity to volunteer for the project. This statement by the Director of the National Service Organization is an attempt to place in the hands of such persons information on the subject.

Volunteers for Project Whitecoat usually are chosen twice a year from among medical soldiers at Fort Sam Houston, Texas. To be eligi-ble for selection a trainee must meet the following criteria:

- be a 1–A–O.

- indicate a preference for the Seventh-day Adventist Church on his religious preference card.

- be assigned to the U.S. Army Medical Training Center.

- not be among those whose names have been sent to the Department of the Army for future assignment.

A selection team from USAMRIID (United States Army Medical Research Institute of Infectious Diseases) screens those who volunteer and chooses those who they feel will best meet the purposes of the project.

Volunteers must be willing to take some risks for a humanitarian cause, but the risk is minimal due to the high degree of protection built into the operation of the project. These details are explained in the lengthy briefing session prior to the individual interviews. During this interview a man may freely express his desire to volunteer or not to volunteer for the project.

Because of their well-known humanitarian ideals, those with a preference for the Seventh-day Adventist Church were chosen as a group from which volunteers could be obtained. Through the years of the project's operation it has had a high degree of performance and low incidence of disciplinary action.

Inasmuch as one of the criteria for selection is a preference for the Seventh-day Adventist Church, it is proper to ask whether the church encourages its members to volunteer for Project Whitecoat. The SDA Church neither encourages nor discourages anyone in volunteering. This is definitely an individual decision to be made on the basis of the information available at the time. If after volunteering and being accepted for Project Whitecoat a man wishes to change his mind and leave the project he can indicate to the Commanding Officer his desire to quit and he will be transferred immediately.

At this point it should be stated that although most persons feel that a great humanitarian service is performed by those in Project Whitecoat, there are some in the church, and elsewhere, who question the basis of the project. The background of the project needs to be understood in this situation.

The organization now known as USAMRIID came into being following the Korean War when two situations developed, either of which could have influenced the formation of the project. Each person will have to choose for himself which of the two was the basis.

First was the fact that during the Korean War U.S. Army hospitals in Korea had several times as many patients from infectious diseases as from actual war inflicted wounds. Many of these infectious diseases were those not normally found in the United States. Americans had not been exposed to these diseases endemic in Korea and had not developed a natural immunity to them. No large research program to develop vaccines of treatment for these diseases had been undertaken such as is the case for those diseases normally found in the United States. It was widely felt that American soldiers subject to service throughout the world should be medically protected against diseases not normally present in the United States but which they might encounter elsewhere. This is the stated reason for the establishment of USAMRIID and accepted as the basis for the project by most people.

The second situation was that the potential of Biological Warfare (BW) was being studied at the same time. Project Whitecoat was not connected with BW by anyone until some fifteen years after the project's establishment. About 1967–68 an upsurge of interest in Chemical and Biological Warfare prompted several persons to write in this field. It was stated that in Biological Warfare a nation must be able to immunize its own personnel against the biological agent to be used in the field so that they will not be effected (sic) by it. When this principle became generally known various persons began to say that Project Whitecoat must have been established with this purpose in view. If this were true then all results of research in developing vaccines, etc. would have been kept a closely guarded secret. Instead, results of research from Project Whitecoat have been published in the professional medical journals of the world.

These are the two situations. Which explanation you choose to accept is completely up to you. The National Service Organization of the SDA church only wants you to be aware of what is being said. The church urges you to ask all the questions you wish before deciding to volunteer or not to volunteer. This is your decision and not the decision of the church. The representative of the SDA Church is here not to take part in the selection process, but to sit in as an interested onlooker in a situation where its members are concerned.

Should you choose to volunteer for Project Whitecoat there are a number of questions that you may have about the SDA Church in the immediate area where those in the project are assigned. The HQ for USAMRIID is Fort Detrick at Frederick, Maryland, some 40 miles north of Washington, D.C. About half of Project Whitecoat participants are assigned there. Most of the others are assigned at Walter Reed Army Hospital in Washington, D.C. or nearby. At both places there are Adventist churches nearby. This is especially so in the Washington, D.C. area where more than a dozen Adventist churches are located. There is also a college (Columbia Union College), a hospital (Washington Sanitarium and Hospital), the General Conference headquarters, and the Review and Herald Publishing Association.

Of more particular interest to men in the Army there is an Adventist servicemen's center in Washington. There are accommodations for sixty to seventy servicemen at this center in a beautiful park-like setting near the college and hospital.

For those servicemen who are married there are apartments near Fort Detrick and near Walter Reed Army Hospital. These are in many price ranges. The pastor at Frederick and the civilian chaplain at the Washington Servicemen's Center can give you some help in locating a place to live. Both in Frederick and in Washington there are normally many job opportunities for those wives who wish to work.

At Columbia Union College and other colleges and universities at both Frederick and Washington, D.C. there are excellent opportunities to take school work on the part of those whose duty hours so permit. Naturally, Army duty comes first in such circumstances.

THE CHURCH & THE MILITARY

The Civil War Years

The Adventist Church originated in the turbulent second and third quarters of the Nineteenth Century, which was a time of great political, economic, social and religious ferment in the United States. The pioneer Adventist leaders by diligent effort, serious Bible study, prayer, and much debate formulated their theological concepts and resultant practices while being influenced by existential factors of the day.

Developing out of the preaching of William Miller and others of the Advent Awakening in the United States, the Seventh-day Adventist Church began in the area of New England and New York. It gradually expanded westward as it established church groups through the upper Midwest and far West. At the time of the Civil War, however, there were no known Seventh-day Adventists anywhere in the States that joined the Confederacy. The Adventist Church developed as a religious movement predicated largely on the belief in the imminent Second Coming of Christ.

As the nation girded itself for the conflict involving the preservation of the Union and the resolution of the slavery question, the youthful Adventist Church experienced traumatic conflict of opinions as to proper courses of action. Later, in 1864, the Church was able to declare that its basic attitude had been "rigidly anti-slavery, loyal to the government and in sympathy with it against the rebellion," as reported in *The Views of Seventh-day Adventists Relative to Bearing Arms* (Battle Creek, MI: Steam Press of the Seventh-day Adventist Publishing Association, 1864 p. 7). This nine-page pamphlet was the first publication of the Church dealing exclusively with noncombatancy.

The vacuum created by the early silence of Church leaders regarding appropriate positions toward involvement in the military and general war effort permitted, if not encouraged, at least three distinct ideologies among both laymen and ministers.

The first view was that slavery must be abolished at any cost and that the Union must be supported, so that participation in such a war was not only justified, but a Christian duty.

The second viewpoint was quite the opposite in that it contended that the Sixth Commandment, "Thou shalt not kill," required total aloofness from all military service in any form in much the same posture as the historic "peace churches," such as the Quakers.

The third ideology contended that it is proper to serve one's nation in any role which does not require bearing of arms, with the individual willing to perform any duty which would relieve him of that responsibility.

The longer the debate went on over the attitude the Church should take about military service, the more the conflicting views seemed to become polarized and rigid (Ellen G. White, *Testimonies for the Church*, vol. 1, Mountain View, CA: Pacific Press Publishing Association 1943, pp. 356–62). The lack of a clarifying statement in *The Review and Herald*, the Church's official publication for its members, did nothing to help those Adventists who were experiencing harassment because they had not come forward and volunteered when President Lincoln had made his call (Arthur Whitfield Spalding, Origin *and History of Seventh-day Adventists*, vol. 1 Washington, DC: Review and Herald Publishing Association, 1962, p. 322). After Congress in 1861 had authorized the President to raise an additional 500,000 troops by voluntary enlistment, various communities had their attention focused on the Adventists as few seem to have volunteered for service.

Various ardent government supporters began to question the patriotism and loyalty of the Adventists so that this became a matter of some embarrassment (White, *op. Cit.*). Thus, in addition to pressures created by the observance of the seventh-day Sabbath, the expectation of the soon return of Christ, and the belief in a woman prophet, was added community concern about the role of Adventists in the war effort. Some among the Adventists who had taken the position of total pacifism publicly announced that they would suffer martyrdom before submitting to the draft, according to Spalding *(op. cit.)*.

The controversy over military service and concern for governmental reaction, combined with fears that the budding church might be wrecked, led James White to publish his editorial, "The Nation," in *The Review and Herald*, August 12, 1862. White apparently intended the editorial to serve as a general statement of the Church on military service and to give guidance to Adventists should they be drafted. Whatever may have been his intention, the editorial led to a heated, extended debate in that paper.

While advancing the arguments that might cause Adventists not to volunteer for military service, James White stressed the patriotism of Adventists and contended that full cooperation with the government was mandatory within all reasonable limits. Writing of the extreme pacifists, he said: "He who would resist until, in the administration of military law, he was shot down, goes too far, we think, in taking the responsibility of suicide. We are at present enjoying the protection of our civil and religious rights, by the best government under heaven. It is Christ-like to honor every good law of our land. Said Jesus, 'Render therefore unto Caesar the things which are Caesar's, and unto God the things which are God's' (ibid.)."

While the Adventist abolitionists argued that the draft would aid God's cause, the pacifists contended that submitting to the draft would automatically violate God's will so that it was unacceptable.

Within two weeks of the appearance of the article, "The Nation," both pacifists and abolitionists were writing to attack it for differing reasons. While perhaps deliberately vague in his editorial, it appears that James White was cautiously advocating Adventists should serve their nation in uniform without bearing arms, while also attempting to keep the Sabbath.

On 3 March 1863, Congress passed the nation's first national conscription law as a means of meeting the requirements of the military. All able-bodied men between 20 and 45 years of age were liable for military service and ordered to enroll with agents of the Provost Marshal General (Fred A. Shannon, *The Organization and Administration of the Union Army, 1861–1865*, Gloucester, MA: Peter Smith, 1928, pp. 305–7). While there were no conscientious objection exemptions, there were two provisions by which a conscriptee could escape military service. He could either furnish a substitute or he could buy an exemption for three hundred dollars.

The Adventists, as a whole, welcomed these legal loopholes as "providential means of avoiding combat services and conflicts over Sabbath observance" (W. C. White, D. E. Robinson, and A.L. White, *Spirit of Prophecy and Military Service*, unpublished manuscript, Ellen G. White Publications, Washington, DC, 1956. p. 13).

In February 1864, an amendment to the conscription law provided that conscientious objectors be regarded as noncombatants when drafted. In these instances, they were to be assigned in hospitals or in caring for freedmen. The Adventists welcomed this amendment, as this provision would permit noncombatant status while serving the nation in military service without violation of convictions against bearing arms. However, recognizing problems inherent in the military for Adventists, they continued to use the commutation procedures as this appeared to be the best plan. Then on 4 July 1864, Congress amended the conscription law by eliminating the option of commutation except for recognized conscientious objectors.

The Years 1866–1920

The Indian Wars, extending from 1817 to 1898, never posed serious questions of sufficient manpower, as the whole series of military actions during that 81 years involved only some 106,000 servicemen. The briefness of the subsequent Spanish-American War of 1898 also never required great masses of military servicemen. There is little, if any, reference to be found in secular newspapers or Church papers about conscription during this period of time. The military needs seem to have been easily met by the regular armed forces in addition to volunteers such as Teddy Roosevelt's Rough Riders.

By October 1916 the General Conference leaders were considering the advisability of defining "our attitude as a denomination on the question of war" (North American Division Annual Conference Committee Minutes, October 15,1916. pp. 424–25). The prevailing consensus was that it was "an inopportune time to make any pronouncements on this question." Nevertheless some leaders, anticipating that the United States would enter the war "suggested that in view of what may be expected in the future, our young men should be given special training in first aid and in caring for the sick."

Some viewed this training as an ideal preparation for renewing the noncombatant status of the Church should United States participation in the war become a reality. Having appointed a subcommittee to study the question of providing pre-military induction training to qualify Adventist Church members for noncombatant duties, the General Conference Committee accepted its five-point program. The three points most relevant to this study were:

1. That more of our young men be encouraged to take the regular nurses courses in our sanitariums' training schools;

2. That as far as consistent there be given in connection with our colleges, particularly to the young men, instruction in simple treatments, fundamental principles of nursing, and "first aid" to the injured, in short such instruction as in times of emergencies will enable them to render service;

3. That a suitable certificate stating the character of this instruction be issued by the Medical Department of the North American Division Conference to those completing this course of instruction.

This series of actions by the General Conference Committee may be the first time any American church seriously attempted systematically to prepare its members for military service prior to actual induction. The foregoing recommendations and actions were a foreshadowing not only of future World War I Seventh-day Adventist Church actions, but a concept which would eventually become the Medical Cadet Program. This program, developed in the 1930's, was a God-sent blessing to thousands of Adventist men during World War II, the Korean War, and the Vietnam War. Indeed, the junior author (DMM) attended Medical Cadet Corps training at Camp Desmond Doss during the Summer of 1967, after registering for the draft, and greatly appreciated the training, as well as the experiences related by Adventist combat medics just returned from Vietnam.

By the spring of 1917, courses in basic nursing and first aid had become part of the Adventist colleges curricula (General Conference Committee Minutes, September 1917, p. 643). Even if these efforts were entirely financed by the Church, and therefore might well be interpreted as efforts to influence governmental officials toward approval of the noncombatant stance of Seventh-day Adventists, basic concepts were formulated that would be later utilized in the Medical Cadet Program.

Although war was declared on 2 April, 1917, the Selective Services Act was not passed by Congress until 18 May, 1917. Even then, the official noncombatant duties were not outlined by President Wilson until 20 March, 1918. On 5 June, 1917 some 9,586,508 young Americans registered for the draft. Of those eventually inducted, only 3,989 claimed exemption on the basis of conscientious objection. This number included those who were willing to serve as noncombatants, of which 450 were pacifists. There appears to be no accurate record of the number of Seventh-day Adventists who were drafted.

As the American government increased its military strength to break the 1918 summer stalemate in Europe, there was a number of Adventist draftees who asserted total pacifism and contended this to be Church-taught. Several were court-martialed for taking a position not permitted by the government. According to one court-martial record (No. 123227), maintained at the Federal Record Center, Suitland, Maryland, the individual received a sentence of 25 years at hard labor for refusing to take the oath and disobeying an order.

Court-martial experiences printed in Adventist literature were obviously for a definite purpose. They tended to be less than representative of a total picture because federal records do not mention just how these convicted conscientious objectors fared. Even the best possible treatment in Fort Leavenworth or Alcatraz would leave much to be desired. Without doubt some men were mistreated by being beaten, put on bread and water diets, intentionally kept awake for extended periods, and needlessly harassed. While always fighting for understanding and fair treatment of its members, the Church leadership struggled to educate members in how to avoid needless difficulties *(The Review and Herald,* July 18, 1918, pp. 4–5; August 1, 1918, pp. 6–7; September 5, 1918, p. 4; and October 17. 1918, p. 16)

With the armistice, on 11 November 1918, most war-service problems ceased for Seventh-day Adventists, except for those who had been court-martialed and were still serving sentences. Newton D. Baker, Secretary of War, permitted all noncombatant prisoners to re-enlist and then to receive honorable discharges. By persistent activity on the part of the Church's Charles Longacre and the federal government's Doctor Keppel, the men in Leavenworth were released by the end of May 1919 with less than honorable discharges.

Unlike the Civil War, which had threatened the Adventist movement as it became a Church, the problems of World War I were largely personal. Moreover, the Adventist Church had been able to renew its governmental recognition of noncombatancy and had developed a methodology of pre-induction training which won admiration, praise and respect from some military officials. In like manner, the Church leadership had learned through experience the wisdom of centrally coordinated Church efforts when dealing with the government. In addition, the selection and utilization of full-time "camp pastors" as on-the-spot observers and counselors to individuals as well as to military commands proved invaluable.

The Years 1920–1939

With the end of World War I, waves of isolationism and pacifistic policies swept over many of the American churches. Some of the more popular American churches that had condemned war and had been quite pacifistic prior to 1914 had undergone a rapid transformation and had ardently supported the war's activities. Now they turned back to their earlier views with renewed ardor in an effort to blot out memories of the Great War.

However, the Seventh-day Adventist General Conference Committee consistently held to the principles inherent in the statement prepared in the 1923 Council of the European Division Committee, meeting in Gland, Switzerland concerning the right of individual freedom of conscience:

In peace and in war we decline to participate in acts of violence and bloodshed. We grant to each of our church members absolute liberty to serve their country, at all times and in all places, in accord with the dictates of their personal conscientious conviction (reported in *The Review and Herald*, March 6, 1924).

Even as this issue was a topic for thought and debate, two events occurred that were mileposts in the Adventist Church, although the first one attracted no attention at the time. In fact, it has been generally unknown and unrecorded in the annals of Adventist Church history. The first was the beginning of the Adventist military chaplaincy in the U.S. Army by Pastor Virgil P. Hulse. The second, was the beginning of the Medical Cadet Program at Union College, under the leadership of Doctor Everett Dick.

Virgil Perry Hulse, the first Seventh-day Adventist minister to hold a commission as an Army chaplain was born 6 February 1896. He had served as a missionary from 1918 to 1922 and as a pastor in the United States from 1922 to 1931. at which time he became a chaplain on duty with the Civilian Conservation Corps (CCC). As a chaplain with the CCC, he submitted monthly reports to the Army Chief of Chaplains, as he was a commissioned Army chaplain and officer subject to all Army regulations and procedures. Apparently in that day the fact of ordination was sufficient evidence for the Army to accept him as a chaplain without the present requirement of ecclesiastical endorsement. Hulse remained on duty until retirement in 1956 as a Colonel.

The establishment, development, and acceptance of the Medical Cadet Program by the Seventh-day Adventist Church was no accident, an action having been taken by the General Conference Committee in 1916 that Adventist colleges provide for the young men of the Church "instruction in simple treatments, fundamental principles of nursing and first aid to the injured...." The purpose of this action was stated thusly: "...[so that] in emergency [the training] will enable them to render service."

The General Conference voted funds to be utilized for barracks for these Institutes of Wartime Nursing (General Conference Minutes, September 26, 1918, p. 135, and November 7, 1918, p. 164). In a way, these actions foreshadowed what would occur during World War II when the Church would strive to provide pre-induction training for any potential draftee willing to undergo a brief, intensive period of indoctrination in military courtesy, drill, and field first aid. To some degree the military drill instructions developed out of the experience of World War I, when it was discovered that such knowledge was most helpful to the Adventist servicemen.

Thus a gathering of various individuals in Denver, Colorado in 1927 urged that some military instruction be given along with paramedical training. This was what Emmanuel Missionary College (now Andrews University) had begun in 1927, only to discontinue it in 1929 because some viewed it as being "too militaristic."

Union College, in Lincoln, Nebraska, was among the Adventist colleges in 1917 to incorporate first aid courses and nursing within their curricula. In view of the political climate in Europe in the early 1930's, members of the Union College faculty discussed in their classes world conditions and appropriate positions toward what might happen. By 1933 the topic of military service was of major interest (Everett N. Dick, *Union: College of the Golden Cords*, Lincoln, NB: Union College Press, 1967, pp. 314–15).

After an unsuccessful attempt to get the Missionary Volunteer Department of the General Conference to lead a discussion of the subject in the 1933 Autumn Council meeting in Battle Creek, Michigan, the President of Union College, M. L. Andersen, led his faculty to establish a study committee composed of faculty members who had been in World War I, with Everett Dick as chairman.

This committee developed the concept and plan for a paramilitary/paramedical service modeled on the military's training system, and having secured the cooperation and approval of appropriate entities, implemented the College Medical Corps.

It met for the first time on the first Monday of January 1934. By the fall of 1934 an advanced grade of training had been developed and implemented. An *esprit de corps* developed before long, and the unit chose an "acceptable uniform." This spirit had as much to do with the success of the project as any other factor.

As the concept spread through the Church, programs were established outside the college environment so that the first name, College Medical Corps, gave way to Medical Cadet Corps, which was the name of a west coast Adventist unit that had received endorsement by the Army Surgeon General for "the training of men as non-commissioned officers." This Corps began training on 26 July, 1936 with 84 individuals led by Cyril B. Courville, an Adventist neurosurgeon and Army Reserve Medical Officer. Doctor Courville's unit was named Medical Cadet Corps, as he envisioned that some trainees would become cadet officers.

The course ran for thirty-four Sundays, with several hours spent each time the class met. The atmosphere generally reflected a disciplined military environment quite similar to Army life of that time (Cyril B. Courville, *Medical Military Training for Civilians*, Arlington, CA: Collegiate Press, 1937, p. 164), and proved sufficiently popular that by the end of 1940 twelve other training units had been established in the Pacific Union Conference.

Meanwhile, Everett Dick won admiration for his Union College unit and other educators wanted similar programs. Expanding the program, Dick held summer courses for non-college students in 1939 and 1940, with a total enrollment of about 125 young men. These summer courses led to the establishment of brief, but intensive summer camps for noncombatant training, in that on 15 October 1939 the General Conference Committee in Autumn Council voted to accept the program for the entire denomination.

The Years 1940–1998

The decade 1940–1950, marked by World War II, was a decisive time for the North American Division of the General Conference in its relationship to the United States Armed Forces. Although records of this period are extant, few scholars or Church administrators are fully aware of the dynamics of change.

While officially neutral in 1939 and 1940, the United States government began to prepare for unavoidable involvement in the War in Europe, which had begun on 1 September 1939 when Germany invaded Poland and England decided that military force must be utilized in order to stop the encroachment of Nazi Germany. A significant step—which clearly signaled the United States government's grave concern—was the congressional debate and passage of the Selective Service Law in September, 1940 with implementation to begin almost immediately.

The General Conference Committee, on 16 September, 1940, voted to re-establish the War Service Commission which had been disestablished with the end of World War I after only a year's existence (Seventh-day Adventist Encyclopedia, Washington, DC: General Conference of Seventh-day Adventists, 1966, p. 504).

Prior to 1950 only three Adventist ministers, Virgil Hulse, Floyd Bresee, and W. H. Bergherm, had been military (Army) chaplains, with their endorsements to the military never approved formally by the General Conference. With the election of W. H. Branson as President of the General Conference, the long-standing attitude of the Church toward the military chaplaincy changed. For the first time, the Church actively recruited six Army chaplains.

Then in March 1953, Robert L. Mole, a returned missionary, was commissioned as the first Adventist Navy chaplain. A few months later Christy Taylor was commissioned as the first Adventist Air Force chaplain.

In 1982 the church, seeing the expanding fields of chaplaincy, moved to restructure the scope of overseeing chaplains. The new department, known as Adventist Chaplaincy Ministries, is charged with responsibility for all professional Seventh-day Adventist Chaplains whether they serve in the military, veteran's affairs (VA), campus, health care or correctional settings. The operations and programs of the National Service Organizations still function as they have in the past, but now those functions are part of a much larger picture.

Once the Operation Whitecoat concept received concurrence of the General Conference, the National Service Organization became the coordinators for the Church to the Army for all Operation Whitecoat issues until the end of the military draft. It should be remembered, however, that the concurrence of the Church for Operation Whitecoat was predicated on the Church's concept of the intimate relationship of theology and health.

THE EXPERIMENTS

The following is a brief description of some of the diseases studied during Operation Whitecoat and some of the experiments performed. Since this is not intended to be a tropical medicine text, for those desiring a detailed review of the experimental methods, results, and discussions, please refer to the appendix and the short bibliography following each section.

Q FEVER

Q Fever is not an Army code word, but an the actual name of a disease. It is usually seen in farmers who become infected by inhalation of dust contaminated with the excretions, placentas, or uterine discharges from cattle, sheep, or goats. There was an outbreak among U.S. Army personnel who sought refuge in barns in southern Europe during World War II.

First described in Australia in 1937, it is an acute infectious disease caused by a small microbe, a rickettsia, called *Coxiella burnetii*. An extremely hardy organism, it can live in dried organic material for up to 18 months or in milk or water for more than 3 years.

Another reason for studying Q Fever, as an airborne disease, i.e. one which results from the inhalation of infectious particles, it provided a prototype by which to study the biomedical and physical aspects of other airborne diseases.

The typical symptoms of fever, chills, headache and muscle aches usually start abruptly after a 9 to 20 day incubation period. In about half of all cases, a non-productive cough develops and a chest x-ray will then usually demonstrate a pneumonia. Some patients may develop liver enlargement, jaundice, and abnormal liver function tests. In the majority of patients, the disease resolves spontaneously after 2 to 4 weeks, but its resolution may be hastened with antibiotic therapy.

Outbreaks of Q fever in military personnel have occurred when troops occupied barns, houses, railroad cars, ships or even pastures previously utilized by animals. Because of its potential ability to at least temporarily disable troops in great numbers, it must be carefully considered when planning military operations in endemic areas. While seldom fatal, and then in only individuals having pre-existing disease(s), it can pose a significant problem for military operations which require prompt and complete action for a successful mission.

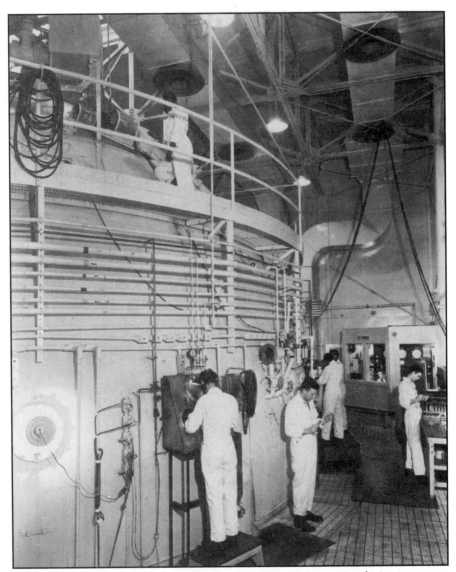

TEST SPHERES- Equator level showing Test Unit Operator in position during a program trial. Left taking Wet and Dry bulb readings at cabinet number 38. Next, taking building humidity reading behind him are two operators at 8BEI cabinet stations. Operator at right with air sampling system. Control room in the background. Upper picture shows 3 level walkway and operator at platform hoist system. (US Army Photo)

After an extensive and successful series of studies in animals, Operation Whitecoat volunteers were exposed in groups to the Q fever disease agent. Each man inhaled a 10-liter sample of aerosol of whole egg slurry containing the infectious organism. The dose given to each group was varied by diluting the infected material with non-infected egg slurry. This mixture was then aerosolized, or made into very small droplets, in the "aerostat" and inhaled by the Whitecoat volunteers. All other exposure factors were held constant. In this way, one would be able to determine what effect the dose, or amount of infectious material inhaled, would have upon the severity of symptoms, the incubation period, and the effectiveness of varying combinations of antibiotics and vaccines.

Also vitally important in the development of protective measures was what droplet size would be of most concern, i.e. be inhaled and remain in the lung tissue to cause infection.

In summary of their report, "Studies on Q fever in man" (*Transactions of the Association of American Physicians*, vol. LXIX, 1956, pp. 98–104), Doctors Tigertt and Beneson stated five findings:

1. *Inasmuch as there is now an effective vaccine against Q fever, the question is, if and when a potentially large population should be immunized against it. Just as the target population can be either military or civilian, is it possible to achieve universal immunization against Q fever?*

2. *Q fever represents only one possible biological enemy or weapon. If thought is given to immunizing target populations, what and how may vaccines are required against all potential agents?*

3. *Inasmuch as the timing of immunization is very important in some infections, when and where should such vaccines be developed, stored and available on short notice, or is this an insurmountable issue at the present time?*

4. *The issue of reactions by differing individuals can be very significant, and may require precautions....Thus what may be highly successful on healthy young adult males may have a different tune when given to children, the aged, the frail, or women in the child-bearing life span.*

5. *Research in Q fever in Project Whitecoat proved that a formalized vaccine of adequate potency is very effective in protecting man and animals against febrile disease. The protection lasts at least 11 months in man and is effective against inhaled doses. Vaccine can be effective in preventing the development of clinical disease if a single dose is administered alter exposure to an aerosol of Q fever provided the challenge is low enough so that the incubation period is sufficiently long for immunity to develop.*

The conclusion was that clinical disease can be averted even after exposure to large doses of *Rickettsiae* if a prophylactic antibiotic is used to prolong the incubation period, and by August of 1958, USAMRIID was able to confidently declare positive results of the Q fever experiments. It stated that the aerosol infectivity of Q fever *Rickettsia* had been determined and the efficiency of a killed vaccine had been achieved in tests against virulent strains. It noted that effective regimens of antibiotic therapy for Q fever in humans were successfully developed. Also, methods were developed for combined use of drug suppression and active immunization for prevention of clinical illness after exposure.

The success of Operation Whitecoat research in Q fever was evident in the Persian Gulf situation in 1990–91 when vaccines prevented Q fever as a major illness and disability in the troops stationed there. Its success is also evident in civilian life for those infected with Q fever.

The major medical and scientific researchers in Q fever were W. D. Tigertt, A.S. Beneson, W.D. Gochenour, Jr. and Joseph Smadel. In many of the references cited hereafter, the authors praise the Seventh-day Adventist draftees who volunteered for this and other medical research programs. The beneficial results will continue for the future even though the names of individuals are not presented.

The following is a partial listing of the researchers' reports to the scientific and medical communities:

U.S. Government Printing Office. TB MED 258, NAVMED P-5052–21 AFP160–5–21 TAGO 1883-A 8 Oct 480468–58 - Q Fever.

W. D. Tigertt and A. S Beneson, "Studies on Q fever in man," *Transactions of the Association of American Physicians*, vol. LXIX, 1956, pp.98–104.

Armed Forces Epidemiological Board Commission of Rickettsial Diseases. *Medical Science Publication No 6, Symposium on Q Fever*, ed. by Joseph E. Smadel, M.D., Walter Reed Army Institute of Research. Washington, DC: Walter Reed Army Medical Center, 1959.

A. S. Beneson, "Q fever vaccine: efficacy and present status," *ibid.*, pp. 47–60. Also in *Military Medicine*, February 1963, pp. 119–28.

Trygve O. Berge, "Public health importance of Q fever," *ibid* pp. 15–19.

William S. Gochenour, Jr., "Veterinary importance of Q fever," *ibid.*, pp. 20–22.

W.D. Tigertt, "Studies on C fever in man," *ibid.*, pp. 34–46.

W.D. Tigertt, "Q fever, in *Current Therapy*," ed. by H.F. Conn. Philadelphia: W B. Saunders, 1960, pp. 35–36.

Dan Crozier, W.D. Tigertt, and Joseph W. Couch, "The physician's role in the defense against biological weapons," *Journal of the American Medical Association*, No. 174, January 7, 1961, pp.4–8.

W.D. Tigertt, Abram [S.] Beneson, and William S. Gochenour, "Airborne Q fever." *Bacteriological Reviews*, vol.25:3, September 1961, pp.285–93.

W.D. Tigertt, "Defensive aspects of biological weapons use," *Military Medicine, vol.* 126:7, July 1961, pp. 502–9.

Dan Crozier, "Military significance of infectious diseases," *Military Medicine*, vol. 127:2, February 1962, pp. 392–96.

Major William D. Sawyer, MC and Phoebe W. Summers, guest editors, "Defense against biological warfare—A symposium," *Military Medicine*, vol. 128:2, February 1963, pp. 81–146.

Robert E. Blount and Dan Crozier, "Antibiotic prophylaxis and treatment," *ibid.*, pp. 129–31.

Dan Crozier, "The threat of biological attack," ibid., pp. 81–85.

Robert W. McKinney, "The laboratory—viral and rickettsial diseases," ibid., p. 102.

W.D. Tigertt, "Status of the medical research effort," *ibid.*, pp. 135–44.

Martha K. Ward. "The laboratory—bacterial and mycotic diseases," *ibid.*, pp. 100–1.

Bernard C. Easterday and Robert F. Jaeger, "The detection of Rift Valley fever virus by a tissue culture fluorescein-labeled antibody method," *Journal of Infectious Diseases*, vol. 112:1, January-February 1963, pp. 1–6.

William R. Beisel and Dan Crozier, "USAMRIID seeks to develop therapy for biological agents," *Army Research and Development Newsmagazine*, vol. 11:7, November-December 1970, pp. 68–69.

Dan Crozier, "The physician and biologic warfare," *New England Journal of Medicine*, vol. 284, May 6, 1971, pp. 1008–11.

R.J. Huebner, W.L. Tellison, W.L. Beck, R.R. Parker, and C.C. Shepherd, "Q fever studies in Southern California, Recovery of *Rickettsia burnetii* from raw milk," *Public Health Reporter*, vol. 63, 1948, pp. 214–22

S.E. Ranson and R. J. Huebner, "Studies on the resistance of *Coxiella burnetii* to physical and chemical agents," *American Journal of Hygiene*, vol. 53, 1951, pp. 110–19.

J.F. Smadel, M.J. Snyder, and F.C. Robbins, "Vaccination against Q fever," *American Journal of Hygiene*, vol.47, 1948, pp. 71–81.

TULAREMIA

Tularemia is a acute fever-producing illness caused by a small bacteria, *Francisella tularensis*. It is especially prevalent in the northern hemisphere with the disease being documented in all of the United States (except Hawaii), Japan, Russia, Canada, and Mexico. Several hundred species of wild animals and insects are known to be naturally infected with the bacteria. Man is most often infected by direct contact with infected meat, especially rabbits, through being bitten ticks or deer flies, or rarely through inhalation of dust or threshings contaminated by moles or other rodents.

Francisella tularensis is a highly virulent microbe with as few as ten organisms known to produce disease in volunteers. The disease produces a highly variable clinic picture, anywhere from a low-grade fever and swollen lymph nodes to a fulminant fatal infection. The usual disease is a sudden onset of fever, chills, headache, backache, malaise, and weakness four or five days after exposure. There are six clinical types of illness, depending upon where the infection entered the body. Before the introduction of antibiotics, the mortality rate was about seven percent. Now it is extremely rare for a treated patient to die.

In awareness of its inherent danger to humans, USAMRIID conducted a number of studies related to tularemia. As previously stated, tularemia acquired by natural means is manifested by a variety of clinical syndromes depending upon the route of infection. Thus one of the primary objectives of the tularemia experiments conducted by McGrumb (Fred R. McGrumb, Jr., "Aerosol infection of man with *Pasteurella (Francisella) tularensis*," Conference on Airborne Infections, Miami Beach, FL, sponsored by Division of Medical Sciences, National Academy of Sciences, National Research Council, December 7–10, 1960, pp. 262–67) and others was to find evidence supporting the idea that respiratory tularemia occurs as a naturally-acquired disease, as well as a deliberately induced disease. Information gained from the study of laboratory-induced disease has led to a much better understanding of the disease producing mechanisms.

It is both interesting and valuable to know that in naturally-occurring instances of respiratory tularemia, the untreated disease, if not fatal, lasts for three to five weeks and is completely disabling.

During World War II hundreds of thousands of the Russian citizens contracted tularemia as a result of a breakdown in public health and sanitation systems. Tularemia has been blamed as a serious cause of disability of the Russian troops on several occasions.

During the course of the Whitecoat experiments designed specifically to assess the effectiveness of vaccines in the prevention of airborne tularemia, the opportunity was present to study the reactions of immunized and non-immunized human beings when exposed to tularemia.

Whitecoat volunteers who were previously vaccinated were exposed to infectious doses varying in size from ten to a thousand times that required to produce disease in humans. Among the subjects, clinically-onset disease appeared within three to five days following exposure to small-particle aerosol. Only the incubation period was affected by the size of the dose received.

All subjects developed full-blown disease characterized by the abrupt onset of fever, headache, chills, sore throat accompanied by malaise, marked myalgia, and backache. Within 24 hours the patients refused food and complained of nausea. Their fevers ranged between 103 and 104 degrees Fahrenheit within the first eight to 24 hours of illness. This phase of tularemia research gave clear evidence tularemia is contracted via the respiratory tract with far greater frequency than had been previously thought.

Other studies conducted by Drs. Shambaugh and Beisel looked at the way in which infections effect blood sugar, i.e. the level of glucose in the blood. It is well known that increased doses of insulin are required in diabetic patients when they are suffering with a infection. In this study, "Insulin response during tularemia in man," a group of seven healthy males with no family history of diabetes nor any prior exposure to synthetic insulin, were given injections of intravenous glucose prior to exposure to tularemia, after the onset of fever, before the start of therapy, and then again two weeks later during convalescence. The rate at which the high levels of injected glucose disappear from the blood stream is an indication of how much insulin is produced by the body, as insulin is required to move the glucose from the blood into the various tissues.

The medical findings clearly suggested that a disturbance in the utilization of glucose my occur very early during clinical illness or even before the onset of fever.

Another group of seven Whitecoat volunteers was also infected with a large dose of *F. tularensis*. Following an incubation period of 24 to 72 hours, illness in the seven patients ranged from a mild headache and malaise without fever to a full systemic response characterized by muscle aches, sensitivity to light, and rectal temperatures reaching 104 degrees Fahrenheit. Patients with fever were treated within 24 hours of the onset of symptoms with streptomycin, one gram twice daily for seven days. Within forty-eight hours of infection and of institution of therapy, patient temperatures became normal and by 72 hours all patients were without symptoms.

The fever-induced clinical illnesses and the changes in glucose tolerance curves, when analyzed statistically, were very similar to those of the first group. This study of insulin and tularemia was an incidental, but not insignificant, part of a continuing long-term series of investigations of vaccine efficiency, diagnostic, and therapeutic methods in infectious disease.

There were also studies involving the effect of artificially raising the body temperature of infected subjects. Only those who had not been vaccinated against the infecting organisms were included. The elevated temperature was induced by raising the temperature and humidity in an environmental chamber. The purpose was to gradually raise the rectal temperature over an 18-hour period to 102.5 degrees F and then maintain that level for six hours, as this was a pattern that mimicked the first day of fever in typical tularemia cases.

Doctor Beisel noted that following the aerosol exposure to *tularensis*, the incubation period generally varied from three to five days and was followed by fever, headaches, malaise and anorexia. Streptomycin therapy at this time reversed the disease process before there could be development of pulmonary findings.

In summary of this very brief overview of USAMRIID's Whitecoat Medical Research experiments regarding tularemia, the following observations are noted:

1. Extensive and extended testing on both animal and man has permitted USAMRIID to determine the maximum infective dose of fully virulent organisms by either injection or respiratory inhalation.

2. Experimentations also demonstrated the decreased infectivity of virulent, aerosolized organisms as their aerosol age increased. This knowledge led to the development of living, attenuated vaccine in Fort Detrick's medical bacteriology laboratory. Found to be both reliable and effective, its use has led to the elimination of tularemia as a laboratory-acquired infection at Fort Detrick and other laboratories.

3. Extensive testing in volunteers proved the vaccine to be fully effective after more than five years of storage. USAMRIID has shared it with other investigators in many other research facilities. In turn, the National Communicable Disease Center has supplied it to numerous research investigators in university settings throughout America.

In addition to the Seventh-day Adventist servicemen who volunteered to participate in the study, the major researchers were T.E. Woodward and R.B. Hornick of the University of Maryland School of Medicine; E.L. Overholt, W.S. Gochenour, Jr., W.D. Tigertt, W.A. Sawyer, P.J. Bartelloni, and Dan Crozier of USAMRIID; and William R. Beisel and Henry T. Eigelsbach from Medical Bacteriology Division, Fort Detrick, Maryland.

The following is a listing of basic references on tularemia:

Edwin L. Overholt and William D. Tigertt, "Roentgenographic manifestations of pulmonary tularemia," *Radiology*, vol. 74:5, May 1960, pp. 758–65.

Robert F. Jaeger, Richard 0. Spertzel, and Ralph W. Kuehne, "Detection of air-borne *Pasteurella-futarensis* using the fluorescent antibody technique," *Applied Microbiology*, vol. 9:6, November 1961, pp. 585–87.

Edwin L. Overholt, William D. Tigertt, Paul J. Kadrell, Martha K. Ward, M. David Charkes, Robert N. Rene, Theodore E. Salzman and Mallory Stephens, "An analysis of forty-two cases of laboratory-acquired tularemia treatment with broad spectrum antibodies," *American Journal of Medicine*, vol.30:5, May 1961, pp. 785–806.

W.D. Tigertt, "Soviet viable *Pasteurella tularensis* vaccines," *Bacteriological Review*, vol. 26:3, September 1962, pp. 354–57.

David Arbiter, "Brain lesions in monkeys infected with *Pasteurella tularensis*," *Journal of Infectious Diseases*, vol. 112:2, May-June 1963, pp.237–42.

William D. Sawyer, Ralph W. Kuehne, and William S. Gochenour, Jr., "Simultaneous aerosol immunization of monkeys with live tularemia and live Venezuelan equine encephalomyelitis vaccines," *Military Medicine*, vol. 129:11, November 1964. pp. 1040–43.

William R. Beisel, Ralph Goldman and Robert J. T. Jay, "Metabolic balance studies during induced hyperthermia in man," *Journal of Applied Physiology, vol.* 24:1, January 1968, pp. 1–10.

Numerous other medical researchers are listed in the above references, some of which are cited below:

Hugh B. Tresselt and Martha K. Ward, "Blood-free medium for the rapid growth of *Pasteurella tularensis.*" *Applied Microbiology.* vol. 12:6, November 1964, pp. 504–07.

U.S. Army Medical Unit Fort Detrick, Maryland, "Studies on *Pasteurella tularensis.*" Section II, Annual Report (358:38082)1958.

William D. Sawyer, Joseph V. Jemski, Arthur Li Hogge, Jr., Henry T. Figelsbock, Elwood K. Wolfe, Harry G. Dangerfield, William S. Gochenour, Jr. and Dan Crozier, "Effects of aerosol age on the infectivity of airborne *Pasteurella tularensis* for *Macaca mulatta* and man," *Journal of Bacteriology*, vol.91:6, June 1966, pp.2180–84.

William D. Sawyer, Harry G. Dangerfield, Arthur L. Hogge and Dan Crozier, "Antibiotic prophylaxis and therapy of airborne tularemia," *Bacteriological Reviews*, vol. 30:3, September 1966, pp. 542–48.

William R. Beisel, "Neutrophil alkaline phosphatase changes in tularemia, sandfly fever Q fever and non-infectious fevers," *Blood*, vol. 29:2, February 1967, pp. 257–68.

William R. Beisel, Joseph Bruton, Kelly D. Anderson and William D. Sawyer, "Adrenocortical and metabolism," vol. 27:1, January 1967,61–69.

W. Sheldon Biven and Arthur L. Hogge, Jr., "Quantitation of susceptibility of swine to infection with *Pasteurella tularensis,*" *American Journal of Veterinary Research*, vol. 28:126, September 1967, pp. 1619–21 .

Ralph D. Feigin and Harry G. Dangerfield, "Whole blood amino acid changes following respiratory-acquired *Pasteurella tularensis* infections in man," *Journal of Infectious Diseases*, vol. 117:4, October 1967, pp. 346–51.

George E. Shambaugh III and William R. Beisel, "Insulin response during tularemia in man," *Diabetes*, vol. 16:6, June 1967, pp. 369–76.

William R. Beisel, Kenneth A. Woeber, Peter J. Bartelloni and Sidney H. Ingbar, "Growth hormone response during sandfly fever," *Journal of Clinical Endocrinology and Metabolism*, vol. 28:8, August 1968, pp. 1220–23.

R.S. Pekarek, Karen A. Bostian, P.J. Bartelloni, F.M. Calia and W.R. Beisel, "The effects of *Francisella tularensis* infection on iron metabolism in man," *American Journal of Medical Sciences*, vol.258:1, July 1969, pp. 14–25.

Harry G. Dangerfield, "Tularemia," in *Current Therapy*. ed. by H.F. Conn, Philadelphia: W. B. Saunders, 1970, pp.69, 70, 200–02.

Martha K. Ward, *"Francisella tularensis,"* in *Manual of Clinical Microbiology*, ed. by John E. Blair, Edwin H. Lennette and Joseph P Truant, Bethesda, Maryland: American Society for Microbiology. 1970, pp. 210–12.

VIRAL ENCEPHALITIS

Viral encephalitis is an infection of the brain tissue. Symptoms include fever, chills, headache, muscle aches, nausea, vomiting, diarrhea and sore throat. In some infections this can progress to confusion, sleepiness, delirium, seizures, coma, and death. Encephalitis can be caused by a number of different viruses—rabies, herpes simplex, herpes zoster, and several types of equine (horse) viruses. Several thousand cases are reported annually in the United States alone. Infection commonly occurs as the result of a mosquito bite, as in the case of the arboviruses, or an animal bite, as in the case of rabies.

The arboviruses are of particular concern since mosquitoes are plentiful in many tropical and semi-tropical areas of the world. The particular type of virus is often named for the area in which it was first discovered and/or the animal, such as the horse, which acts as a reservoir for the disease. Examples include St. Louis Encephalitis, Eastern Equine Encephalitis, Western Equine Encephalitis, Venezuelan Equine Encephalitis.

Venezuelan Equine Encephalitis (VEE) was first recognized along the Venezuela-Colombia border in 1935. But it took an additional three years before the virus was isolated in 1938 from equine brain tissue during another outbreak in Venezuela. The major encephalitis epidemic of 1942 in Venezuela spread to Trinidad, and it was there in 1943 that Colonel Raymond Randall of the Walter Reed Army Institute of Research reported the first isolate from the brain of a human fatality.

In April 1971, VEE cases were being discovered and diagnosed just 250 air miles from Brownsville, Texas in the Tampico region of Mexico. On 10 July 1971 in Live Oak County, Texas, the first case of an animal infected with VEE was confirmed. By 1 September 1971 nearly 1,500 horses in Texas had died and the disease continued marching northward. For statistical purposes a "major outbreak" or "epidemic" occurs when 100 to 1,000 horses are attacked in a given locale. Venezuelan equine encephalomyelitis cases are normally much greater in the hot, summer months when the insect population is highest since the mosquito is the primary transmitter of the disease.

As noted earlier, Colonel Raymond Randall in 1944 reported on the first isolate of VEE from a human brain, and also provided the characterization of an isolate from a donkey brain. These developments began a long journey toward the successful development of an approved VEE vaccine.

Randall's first step was to take the virus isolate of the donkey brain and prepare an inactivated vaccine grown in chicken egg solution. His second major step, in 1949, was to use this vaccine to vaccinate at-risk laboratory personnel who potentially might be exposed to this disease. USAMRIID began to grow the viral strain isolated by Colonel Randall in tissue cultures. After extensive laboratory tests indicated that the live virus, which had undergone numerous laboratory changes, was now hopefully nonvirulent (by having been tested on a large number of laboratory animals, including burros), it was ready for human testing.

The first individual to be officially tested was Colonel T.0. Berge of USAMRIID in 1959. He volunteered and was selected as he already had experienced a laboratory-acquired infection with a virulent VEE virus. After studies on Colonel Berge were satisfactorily completed, the vaccines were then administered to individuals believed partially protected inasmuch as they previously had received inactivated vaccine. As this proved inconclusive, the next major step was to administer this vaccine to five persons who had no previous exposure to either the VEE virus or to the vaccine.

Because the vaccinated individuals developed influenza-like symptoms, more research was essential since the vaccine obviously was not yet suitable for human use. It was determined further weakening of the vaccine's side effects was essential, so studies of virus growth in tissue culture continued. USAMRIID was searching for a living virus that would provide protection but not cause the disease. With the development of weakened virus vaccine, experiments were again done on animals. Having achieved apparent success, the next step was to use the improved vaccine on human volunteers. Enter Operation Whitecoat volunteers.

USAMRIID conducted some 17 different studies on the nature of encephalitis. A total of some 240 Operation Whitecoat volunteers participated after the newly-developed vaccine was standardized in 1961. As the experimental vaccine proved stable, effective, and acceptable for routine administration (at first to laboratory personnel working with virulent strains of VEE virus) its use was broadened.

Routine use of USAMRIID-produced vaccine became the practice in several Army laboratories. It is now available for the commercial market, with National Drug Company of Pennsylvania as the major producer.

Major participants in the VEE research effort, in addition to the Whitecoat volunteers, included T.0. Berge, C.A. Gleiser, W.S. Gochenour, Jr., A.L. Hogge Jr., R.W. McKinney, E.L. Overholt, and Colonel W.D. Tigertt all of USAMRIID; along with Colonel Raymond Randall of the U.S. Army Walter Reed Institute of Research; P.J. Kadull, Medical Investigation Division, Fort Detrick, Maryland; and W. G. Downs, Director of the Trinidad Virus Laboratory, Port of Spain, Trinidad, West Indies.

One experiment reported in the *American Journal of Tropical Medicine and Hygiene*, 1967, was entitled "Live, attenuated Venezuelan equine encephalomyelitis virus vaccine: I. Clinical effects in man," by Aristedes C. Alevizatos, Robert W. McKinney and Ralph D. Feigin (see list of references). In this medical research project, 40 healthy, young Whitecoat volunteers, aged 19 to 26 years, without any prior VEE virus exposure, were participants. All were fully informed of the nature of the project, including details and risks of the study before any actual participation. No one was accepted into the study unless laboratory findings were within accepted normal limits.

Another encephalitis experiment was the use of a formalin-inactivated Eastern Equine Encephalitis (EEE) vaccine, prepared in chick-embryo cell cultures, injected just underneath the skin in 16 volunteers. There were no meaningful changes in clinical laboratory values during the evaluation period, with only mild reactions in some of the volunteers. Serologic responses seemed to indicate that a two-dose series with a 28-day interval would result in significant and persistent protection.

Additional information can be found in the following:

Robert W. McKinney, Trygve 0. Berge, W.D. Sawyer, W.D. Tigertt and Dan Crozier "Use of an attenuated strain of Venezuelan equine encephalomyelitis virus for immunization In man," *American Journal of Tropical Medicine and Hygiene*, vol. 12:4, July 1963, pp. 597ff.

Anstedes C. Alevizatos, Robert W. McKinney, and Ralph Feigin, "Live, attenuated Venezuelan equine encephalomyelitis virus vaccine: I. Clinical effects in man," *The American Journal of Tropical Medicine and Hygiene*, vol. 16:8, 1967; and in the same journal, Ralph D. Feigin, Robert F. Jaeger, Robert W. McKinney, and Aristedes C. Alevizatos, "II. Whole-blood amino acid and fluorescent-antibody studies following immunization."

Louis F. Maire III, Robert W. McKinney and Francis E. Cole, Jr., "An inactivated eastern equine encephalomyelitis vaccine propagated in chick-embryo cell culture: I. Production and testing," *American Journal of Tropical Medicine and Hygiene*, vol., 19:1, January 1970, pp. 119–22. Also in *Arthropod-Borne Virus Information Exchange. vol. 19*, January 1970, pp. 132–34.

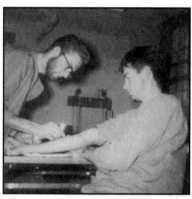

Whitecoat John D. Smith draws blood from fellow Whitecoat Henning Goldhammer during one of the experiments.

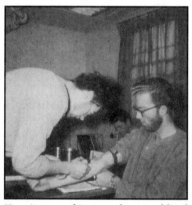

Henning gets his turn drawing blood from John.

Peter J. Bartelloni, Robert W. McKinney, Thomas P. Duffy and Francis E. Cole, Jr., "An inactivated eastern equine encephalomyelitis vaccine propagated in chick-embryo cell culture: II. Clinical and serologic responses in man," *The American Journal of Tropical Medicine and Hygiene*, vol. 19:1, January 1970, pp. 123–126. Also in *Arthropod-Borne Virus Information Exchange*, vol. 19, July 1969, pp. 134–36.

Robert S. Pekarek George A. Berghen, Peter J. Bartelloni, Frank M. Calia, Karen A. Bostian and William R. Beisel, "The effect of live, attenuated Venezuelan equine encephalomyelitis virus vaccine on serum iron, zinc, and copper concentrations in man," *The Journal of Laboratory and Clinical Medicine*, vol. 76:2, August 1970, pp. 293–303.

Peter J. Bartelloni, Robert W. McKinney, Frank M. Calia, Helen H. Ramsburg and Francis E. Cole, Jr., "Inactivated western equine encephalomyelitis vaccine propagated in chick embryo cell culture," *Journal of Tropical Medicine and Hygiene*, vol. 20:1, 1971.

Edward V. Staab and Sigurd J. Normann, "Alternations in reticuloendothelial function by infection with attenuated Venezuelan equine encephalitis (VEE) virus," *Journal of the Reticuloendothelial Society*. vol., 8:4, October1970, pp. 342–48, pp. 146–49.

SANDFLY FEVER

Sandfly fever is a general term used for an acute, self-limited febrile illness which can be caused by more than 38 different viruses. It is seen in tropical areas of the world and, therefore, the history of sandfly fever is closely tied to military campaigns. During World War II almost 20,000 cases were reported among U.S. troops alone.

The insect, Phlebotomus papatasi, is a nocturally biting midge who likes to feed on humans. They breed in organic debris and loose soil near dwellings and are small enough, 2 to 3 millimeters, that they readily pass through screens and mosquito netting.

Symptoms start about three to six days after being bitten and include fever, headache, nausea, vomiting, and body aches. The illness lasts about three days, but is followed by one to two weeks of weakness, fatigue, and depression.

Several experiments were conducted at USAMRIID involving Sandfly Fever and the results can be found in the following scientific articles:

William R. Beisel, "Neutrophil alkaline phosphatase changes in tularemia, sandfly fever, Q fever, and non-infectious fevers," *Blood*, vol., 29:2 February 1967, pp. 257–68.

W. R. Beisel, W. D Sawyer, E. R. Ryll and Dan Crozier in *Annals of Internal Medicine*, vol. 67, 1967, p. 744.

In addition the above sandfly fever research, which had included measurement of work performance during acute tularemia and sandfly fever, another study was done. This one attempted to determine if a brief course of symptomatic therapy could reduce or even eliminate the lower levels of work performance associated with sandfly fever. This was reputed to be the first study of this nature and proved to be quite successful.

The therapy used was 48-hours of aspirin and Darvon, which proved adequate to markedly reduce the fever of the Whitecoat volunteers as well as other symptoms of illness. This therapeutic response was accompanied by the volunteers' ability to sustain a work performance much greater than that of untreated subjects of the experiment.

Other tests of sandfly fever virus infection included one with six infected subjects and another with eight subjects. The results of both studies indicate that measurable biochemical and functional changes occur in some types of white blood cells during the course of a viral infection. The two tests were reported by the researchers, Joseph A. Belloni, Mel C. Yang, Robert I. Krasner, Peter J. Bartelloni and William R. Beisel, at the Annual Meeting of the Federation of American Societies for Experimental Biology.

Operation Desert Storm (also called the Persian Gulf War), in early 1991, demonstrated anew the value of continuing the carefully-controlled and monitored scientific medical research with human volunteers. A number of U.S. troops returned from that war with rare parasitic infections acquired through the bites of sand flies. As of 25 November 1991, some 22 soldiers tested positive for leishmaniasis. In most cases the infection was essentially a localized skin disease, but in seven cases leishmania had invaded the bone marrow and internal organs, according to Colonel Charles Oster, Chief of Infectious Diseases, Walter Reed Army Medical Center.

The main symptoms of leishmaniasis are fever, diarrhea and abdominal pains. In some soldiers, the fever was sudden and high; others developed low, persistent fevers that left them fatigued. Some victims developed enlarged spleens and livers. Some soldiers had no symptoms, but were found to be infected.

Sandfly fever is curable with the drug Pentostom, manufactured in Britain. The drug is administered intravenously for twenty minutes a day by drip infusion. Treatment for skin infections of leishmania takes 20 days, whereas it takes 30 days of daily treatment to kill the parasites when the bone marrow and internal organs are infected.

ROCKY MOUNTAIN SPOTTED FEVER

Rocky Mountain spotted fever (RMSF) is the most common rickettsial disease in the United States. It is one of a group of tick-borne diseases which is on the increase as a result of human migration into rural areas, outdoor recreational activities, and reforestation. Other major tick-borne diseases in the United States include Lyme disease, Tularemia, Ehrlichiosis, Relapsing fever, Colorado tick fever, Babesiosis, and Tick paralysis.

In simple terms, Rocky Mountain spotted fever is an acute infectious disease caused by mosquito bites which produce fever, joint and muscular pains, aversion to light and sometimes delirium, coma, convulsions, tremors, muscular rigidity and jaundice. Persistent effects may include deafness, impaired vision and anemia. The mortality rate in untreated cases averages about 22 percent but can run as high as 80 percent.

Work by USAMRIID in this area can be found in the following:

Frank M. Calia, Peter J. Bartelloni and Robert W. McKinney, "Rocky Mountain spotted fever: Laboratory infection in a vaccinated individual," *Journal American Medical Association*, vol. 211:12, March 1970, pp. 2012–14.

TYPHUS & TYPHOID FEVER

These two diseases are commonly confused, but are caused by completely different organisms. Epidemic typhus fever is a lice or flea-borne disease a cause by a rickettsia, whereas typhoid fever is a bacterial infection caused by *Salmonella typhi*. Some of this confusion can be blamed on a French physician in the early nineteenth century who referred to a "typhus-like" fever as typhoid. Both fevers take their name from the Greek "typhos," meaning smoke, which refers to the apathy and confusion arising from fever.

Typhus is any of a group of related arthropod-borne infectious diseases caused by a species of *Rickettsia* and marked by malaise, severe headache, sustained high fever, and a rash which appears from the third to the seventh day.

Typhoid fever is found in all parts of the world. In the Spanish-American War, about twenty percent of U.S. troops developed typhoid fever and over 1500 died. During the South African Boer War, the British Army lost more men to typhoid fever than it did to war wounds. In 1909 there were half a million cases of typhoid fever and almost ten percent of those died.

For information regarding typhus and typhoid experiments conducted by USAMRIID, consult the following references:

W.D. Tigertt, "The initial effort to immunize American soldier volunteers with typhoid vaccine," *Military Medicine*, vol. 124:5, May 1959, pp. 342–49.

Geoffrey Edsoll, Sidney Gaines, Maurice Landy, W. D. Tigertt, Helmuth Sprinz, R. J. Traponai, Adrian D. Mandel and A. S. Beneson, "Studies on infection and immunity in experimental typhoid fever: I. Typhoid fever in chimpanzees orally infected with *Salmonella typhosa*," *Journal of Experimental Medicine.* vol. 112:1, July 1960, pp. 143-66.

Joseph G. Tully, Sidney Gaines and William D. Tigertt, "Attempts to induce typhoid fever in chimpanzees with non-virulent strains of *Salmonella typhosa,*" *Journal of Infections Diseases,* vol. 110:1, January-February 1962, pp. 47–54.

Joseph G. Tully, Sidney Gaines and William D. Tigertt, "Studies on infection and immunization experimental typhoid fever: IV. Role of H. antigen in protection," *Journal* of Infectious Diseases, vol. 112:2, March-April 1963, pp. 118–72.

Ralph D. Fergin, Albert S. Klainer, William R. Beisel and Richard B. Honnick, "Whole-blood amino acids in experimentally-induced typhoid fever in man," *New England Journal of Medicine,* vol. 278:6, February 8,1968. pp. 293–98.

Dan Crozier, "Typhus fever," in *Current Therapy,* ed. by H. F. Conn. Philadelphia: W B. Saunders, 1960, pp. 72–73.

RIFT VALLEY FEVER

Rift Valley fever is an acute viral infection of livestock and humans in Africa. The infection can range from a flu-like illness to a hemorrhagic (bleeding) fever. It is transmitted by mosquito and outbreaks coincide with periods of heavy rainfall. The disease can also be transmitted by aerosols.

In most cases the patient develops fever, chills, headache, low back pain, loss of appetite, nausea and vomiting. The disease usually runs its course in four to seven days and recovery is complete. In a small number of cases, bleeding disorders and brain infection can result in death.

Rift Valley fever vaccine, formalin inactivated, of tissue culture origin, was developed and tested on volunteers so successfully that it can now be made by large-scale methods. The vaccine has been found to be both safe and immunogenic through studies conducted in animals as well as by serum neutralization tests in volunteers. As noted above, Rift Valley fever is rarely fatal, but is sufficiently disabling to adversely effect economic output. White-coat volunteers were part of the research on vaccine developed for this disease.

More information can be obtained by reading:

Bernard C. Easterday, and Robert F. Jaeger, "The detection of Rift Valley fever virus by a tissue culture fluorescein-labeled antibody method," *Journal of Infectious Diseases,* vol. 112:1 January-February 1963, pp. 1–6.

YELLOW FEVER

Yellow fever is an acute mosquito-borne disease characterized by fever, jaundice (hence the name yellow fever), and hemorrhage. It is endemic and epidemic in tropical regions of the Americas and Africa.

A physician in Havana, Cuba, Dr. Carlos J. Finlay, postulated in 1881 that the disease was transmitted by mosquitoes. U.S. Army Major Walter Reed and his associates proved Finlay's theory at the turn of the century.

For the past 200 years, yellow fever has been responsible for devastating epidemics and massive economic losses. Yellow fever continues to be a major problem with 100,000 cases reported annually in Africa alone. Fatalities occur in about thirty percent of untreated cases. While the mechanism is not completely understood, the virus causes injury to major target organs, usually the liver. Fatal cases present with hepatitis, hemorrhage, and shock.

Recognizing the inherent danger and effects of yellow fever, and in awareness that Americans may be required to serve in yellow fever-endemic areas, effective medical knowledge and preventive or therapeutic technology are essential. Moreover such knowledge applied to indigenous peoples can greatly reduce illness and misery for them.

Whitecoat volunteers were involved in a USAMRIID study of certain human metabolic and immunologic responses involving the administration of a 17-D strain of yellow fever vaccine.

The 17-D strain of yellow fever vaccine tends to create a mild infection in humans but has proven to be a safe vaccine with few clinical reactions. Research has shown that five to 10 percent of those vaccinated develop mild headaches, myalgia, low grade fever, and/or other mild symptoms from five to 10 days after vaccination.

Incidentally, the Whitecoat volunteers were in strict isolation except for access by clearly defined researchers and hospital staff, and were able to choose either a regular house diet or vegetarian diet.

In order to be as scientifically accurate as possible, the study specified who might come into the volunteer wards. This list included: Commanding Officer, Principal Investigators, Ward Officer Chief of Nursing Service, and Chief of the Pathology Division, all of whom would designate in writing their personnel who were to be admitted to the wards, with the Chief Medical Officer serving as approving official. No one with any illness of any type was admitted.

Maintenance personnel were authorized only by Chief of Nursing Service responsible for maintaining discipline, with any infractions to be immediately reported to the Chief of the Medical Division. In spite of the restrictions, patient care took precedence over investigational procedures.

With COL Dan Crozier, MC, as the project director, the principal investigators of this study were Peter J. Bartelloni, LTC, MC; Robert W.

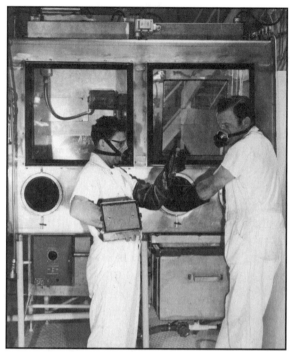

Isolation Facility for handling highly infectious materials.
US Army Photo

Wannemacker, Jr., Ph.D.; Robert S. Pekarek, Ph.D.; and Albert T. McManus, CAPT, Medical Service Corps.

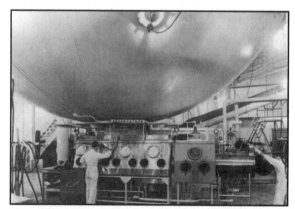

The aerostat was designed to test the size of particles that carry infectious materials which are inhaled.

(US Army Photo)

PLAGUE

Plague, the "Black Death," has profoundly effected western civilization socially, culturally, and economically. Three major pandemics of bubonic plague have been recorded since the birth of Christ. One fourth the population of Europe is estimated to have died as the result of this disease caused by *Yersinia pestis*. A Swiss bacteriologist, Alexandre Yersin, was able to isolate the bacteria from dead victims during an epidemic in Hong Kong in 1894. By obtaining pure cultures of the organisms, he was able to demonstrate its lethal effect in experimental animals, thereby establishing a cause-effect relationship.

The plague is carried by rodents and is transmitted to humans by bites from infected fleas. Mortality is high in untreated cases, but fortunately the disease responds well to antibiotics.

According to reports of USAMRIID studies in both humans and animals, killed plague vaccine provides substantial protection against virulent *Y. pestis*. This observation is based upon the measured production of antibodies in humans, and in animals by their survivability.

USAMRIID engaged in a year-long evaluation of the serological responses of Whitecoat volunteers to the administration of Plague Vaccine, U.S.P. (E. Medium). Some 29 Whitecoat volunteers received 1.0 ml of plague vaccine on day 0, followed on day 90 and day 270 by 0.2 ml booster doses of the vaccine. Blood drawn for serological studies was obtained at various intervals both before and after vaccination.

The conclusion, reached in 1970 after nine months of experimentation, was that the present plague immunization program provides considerable protection against flea-borne plague infections.

Additional information may be obtained by reading the following:

D.C. Cavanaugh, P.J. Deoras, D.H. Hunter, J.D. Marshall, Do-Van-Quy, J. H. Rust, Jr., Sithibun Purnaveja and P. E. Winter, "Some observations on the necessity for serological testing of rodent sera for *Pasteurella pestis* antibody in a plague control programme." *Bulletin, World Health Organization* vol.42:3, March 1970, pp. 451–59.

VACCINE COMBINATIONS

One of the more challenging scientific medical research programs has been developing a method of combining vaccines or administering them simultaneously in order to shorten vaccination schedules without producing toxicity or loss of the effectiveness of each vaccine in the combination.

Vaccines for Eastern Equine Encephalitis (EEE) and Western Equine Encephalitis (WEE) administered as a combined vaccine in man was found to effective with an adequate production of antibodies. This study, performed on Whitecoat volunteers, included the administration of a combined EEE and WEE vaccine administered simultaneously with a living Venezuelan equine encephalomyelitis vaccine at a different site. There were no unanticipated reactions, so antibody responses to all three vaccines were accepted as satisfactory.

In 1970, in preparation for future testing of combined vaccines, the efficiency of a pentavalent vaccine composed of EEE and WEE, Rift Valley fever, chikungunya, and Q fever vaccines was determined in animals. It was discovered that each component of the combined vaccines was as effective as if it were used alone. Inasmuch as the medical research was focused on human beings, procedures for its acceptability in human use required ongoing testing and evaluation.

HYPERTHERMIA

Lieutenant Colonel William R. Beisel also did medical research utilizing Operation Whitecoat participants to study "Metabolic and endocrine effects of infection and hyperthermia" (see list of references). The metabolic studies were conducted on a large group of Whitecoat volunteers who were exposed to either an aerosol of *Pasteurella tularensis* or to artificial hyperthermia.

Hyperthermia, induced by a hot humid environment, invoked many physiologic responses quite different from those seen in reactions to infections. Yet the similarities of many observed changes suggested that fever, by and of itself, is a contributing factor for metabolic changes associated with acute infections.

During these studies, some volunteers were exposed to highly infectious and/or to partially attenuated organisms. Others were exposed after immunization against *Pasteurella tularensis;* still others after a recent previous episode of acute tularemia; and as an additional control two men were sham-exposed. An additional effort to differentiate the metabolic effects of hyperthermia alone led to an experiment of induced fever in one group while on the metabolic balance study. To do this, it was necessary to use a hot and humid environment to reproduce the febrile response typical of the disease.

The physically-induced hyperthermia was brought about gradually and lasted only a single day. Body temperature during the final six hours was maintained no higher than 102.5 degrees Fahrenheit (taken rectally). Even so, there were marked changes in metabolism.

The conclusion of these studies was that hyperthermia induced by moist external heat presents both similarities and differences in metabolism as seen in patients with infections. According to Doctor Beisel, these studies were the first reported attempt to survey metabolic changes in the normal host during induced infection in a broad, systematic and prospective fashion.

For a more detailed explanation see:

Symposium on Medical Aspects of Stress in the Military Climate, "Metabolic and endocrine effects of infection and hyperthermia," 22–24 April 1964, Washington, D.C., Walter Reed Army Institute of Research, 1965, pp. 523–37.

William R. Beisel, Ralph F. Goldman and Robert J. T. Joy, "Metabolic balance studies during induced hyperthermia in man." *Journal of Applied Physiology*, vol. 24:1, January 1968, p. 10.

USAMRIID directed, and continues to direct, major efforts toward development of rapid diagnostic measures and appropriate treatment for infectious diseases. Research has revealed that the most prominent, infection-related metabolic responses of the infected host begins in conjunction with the onset of symptomatic illness and are generally proportional in magnitude to both severity and duration of the disease. It is remarkable that in all symptomatic bacterial, viral and rickettsial infections, similar patterns of nitrogen, electrolyte and mineral losses from tissue are produced.

The broad medical research program of USAMRIID provides data upon which more specific defensive medical measures can be based. USAMRIID served, and continues to serve, all of medicine by contributing to a fundamental understanding of infectious diseases along with prevention and treatment modalities. This is well explained in an article by William R. Beisel and Dan Crozier, "USAMRIID seeks to develop therapy for biological agents," *Army Research and Development Newsmagazine*, November-December 1970. pp. 68–69.

The medical research experiments previously listed, as well as many others, are part of an ongoing endeavor to understand and prevent infectious disease. The utilization of human volunteers as experimental subjects under carefully controlled and monitored conditions has, and does, greatly enhance the rapidity with which new vaccines become available for use both in America and around the world.

The entire research program of this organization is unclassified and all information accruing from these studies is reported, as appropriate, in the medical literature. Thus the results of the total effort in the Army research program in medical defense against biological weapons is made available to the scientific world.

In addition to the published reports previously referenced, the following are sources of additional information:

D.A. Rhoda, D.D. Elsberry and W.R. Beisel, "Fluid compartment alterations in the monkey with staphylococci B enterotoxemia," *American Journal of Veterinary Research*, vol. 31:3. March 1970, pp. 507–14.

Jerry S. Walker, James D. Rundquist, Rodney Taylor, Byron Lee Wilson, Michael R. Andrews, John Barck, Arthur L. Hogge, Jr., David L. Huxsoll, Paul K. Hildebrandt and Robert M. Nims, "Clinical and clinicopathologic findings in tropical canine pancytopenia," Journal *American Veterinary Medical Association*, vol.157:1, July 1970, pp. 43–55.

William R. Beisel and Robert H. Fiser, Jr., "Lipid metabolism during infectious illness," *American Journal of Clinical Nutrition*, vol. 23:8, August 1970, pp. 1069–79.

J. Brent Rollins, Charles H. Hobbs, Richard 0. Spertzel and Stewart McConnell, "Hematologic studies of the rhesus monkey *(Macaca mulatta)," Laboratory Animal Care*, vol. 20:4, August 1970, pp. 681–85.

M.I. Rapoport, W.R. Beisel and R.B. Hornick, "Tryptophan metabolism during infectious illness in man," *Journal of Infectious Diseases*, vol. 122:3, September 1970, pp. 159–69.

D.A. Rhoda and W.R. Beisel, "Lymph production during staphylococcic B enterotoxemia-induced shock in monkeys," *American Journal of Veterinary Research*, vol. 31:10, October 1970, pp. 1845–51.

J. Brent Rollins, George A. Burghen and William R. Beisel, "The influence of altered viral virulence on the response of host serum alpha-2 glycoglobulins," *Journal of Infectious Diseases*, vol. 122:4, October 1970, pp. 329–34.

George A. Burghen, William R. Beisel and Peter J. Bartelloni, "Influences of chloramphenicol administration on whole blood amino acids in man," *Clinical Medicine*, vol. 77:11, November 1970,-29.

Michael C. Powanda and Robert W. Wannemacher, Jr., "Evidence for a linear correlation between the level of dietary tryptophan and hepatic NAD concentration and for a systematic variation in tissue NAD concentration in the mouse and the rat," *Journal of Nutrition*, vol. 100:12, December 1970, pp. 1471–78.

John D. Marshall, Jr., and Daniel C. Kavanagh *"Pasteurella,"* Chapter 20 in *Manual of Clinical Microbiology*, ed. by John E. Blair, Edwin H. Linette and Joseph P. Truant, Bethesda, Maryland: American Society for Microbiology, 1970, pp. 205–09.

THE CHURCH REVIEWS ITS PARTICIPATION

The late 1960's and 1970's was a period of turbulence and social unrest in America. Almost all institutions and concepts of moral and social responsibility were under attack. Traditional Church teachings and practices were being strongly criticized. An unpopular war in Vietnam, political assassinations, abuse of power by high government officials, worsening economic conditions, and the disclosure of government secrets created a general feeling of mistrust of those in authority. Anyone in the military, or associated closely with it, was suspect in the minds of large segments of the American populous. In addition, it is a long standing American tradition to have a healthly distrust of government. Otherwise, the Founding Fathers would not have included the Second Amendment to the Constitution or reserved the right to alter or abolish government should it become tyrannical or despotic.

Without the benefit of a careful examination of the reasons, objectives, or results, cooperative programs between the Seventh-day Adventist Church and the military were deemed evil by some observers. Much of the argument against harmonious, cooperative church-military relations was made with little knowledge or awareness of the historical traditions and practices of either the Church or the American military.

After Operation Whitecoat had been in progress for more than a decade, it became a source of rather bitter polemics by those who objected to it. Media coverage of the Vietnam era both in Vietnam and in America tended to portray the U.S. government as intrinsically evil in thought and deed. Thus it was that critics in the media and on Adventist college campuses encouraged church officials to review the program. Before detailing how Adventist leadership responded in 1969, it would be useful to point out how the military perceived Operation Whitecoat.

The following statement was given to each soldier volunteering for Operation Whitecoat while at Fort Sam Houston. Only those who signed up for the Project were interviewed. According to Army officials, only about one in three of the volunteers was selected, as the Army limited the number because of restrictions imposed by higher authorities.

For Use at Fort Sam Houston, Texas

A program of investigation conducted by the United States Army Medical Research Institute of Infectious Diseases, Fort Detrick, Maryland, has been explained to me. I understand that this program consists of studies dealing with various aspects of infectious diseases,

including nature of the infection, diagnosis, prevention, and treat-
ment, and that studies in volunteers are essential for a complete
evaluation of these processes. I further understand that such volun-
teers may become ill and that the program is not without hazard.

My signature below indicates my desire to participate in PRO-
JECT WHITECOAT to be assigned to the United States Army Medical
Research Institute of Infectious Diseases, and to participate in these
volunteer studies, with the following three provisos:

1. *That prior to the actual conduct of a study, full details of my*
   part in the program will be given to me;
2. *That after this more detailed explanation, I may withdraw*
   from the study without prejudice; and
3. *That I will not be required to participate in studies which, in*
   themselves, are contrary to my religious or moral precepts.

After being chosen as a Whitecoat volunteer and reporting to
the appropriate medical command at either Walter Reed Army Hospital or Fort Detrick, an additional research agreement was utilized. At the time an actual research project had been approved and
was ready to be operational, only those who had signed the following agreement were accepted for that particular research project.

DEPARTMENT OF THE ARMY

U.S. ARMY MEDICAL RESEARCH INSTITUTE OF INFECTIOUS
DISEASES

FORT DETRICK

FREDERICK, MARYLAND 21701

CONSENT STATEMENT

I _____, without duress and of my own free will do
hereby consent to participate in a research study conducted by physi-
cians of the U.S. Army Medical Research Institute of Infectious Dis-
eases, Fort Detrick, Frederick, Maryland involving
_____.

The implications of such a study have been explained to me. I under-
stand that an element of risk is involved in this procedure.

I understand that this is an approved research study and as such will be recorded in official files of the Department of the Army. Any medical problems arising from my participation in this study will be considered to have been incurred in the line of duty. I also understand that no additional rights against the government will accrue from my having participated as a volunteer.

In addition to the foregoing acknowledgments, a detailed "Research Data Record" (SMUFD Form 2027) was kept on each Whitecoat volunteer by the Medical Division of USAMRIID; each person had a record whether or not he had ever been "on the project." The Administrative Division of USAMRIID also kept an "In-Processing and Locator Record" (WRAMC Form 59), which was a detailed record of personal information on each volunteer.

In February 1968, Pastor Theodore Carcich, Chairman of the National Service Organization Committee and Vice President of the General Conference of Seventh-day Adventists said of Project Whitecoat in the NSO Chaplain School Manual, pp. 27–28:

PROJECT WHITECOAT

There is a well-known volunteer program which Seventh-day Adventist l–A–0 draftees enter, entitled Project Whitecoat. Though composed of SDA volunteers, this is not a program operated by the church. This is an Army program. The reason the volunteers are all Adventist 1–A–0's is a practical situation for the military. In any volunteer program in the military, all who wish to enter such a program, must be given an opportunity to do so if they are in the group from which volunteers will be taken. To simply open Army-wide the opportunity to volunteer for this program would immediately engulf the officers selecting the volunteers in a mass of applications, all of which must be given equal opportunity. Thus the program of drastically narrowing the field from which volunteers would be obtained simplifies their problem. The only thing is that they must be certain to have a large enough group from which to get their required numbers.

Thus far the Adventist 1–A–O draftees in training at Fort Sam Houston Medical Training Center (Basic or AIT) have provided a rich group for selecting the number necessary to maintain the volunteer group strength. A selection team goes to the Medical Training Center twice a year and chooses the number necessary to keep their author-

ized strength at 175. The exact dates for these two visits per year are never set until approximately six weeks prior to the time.

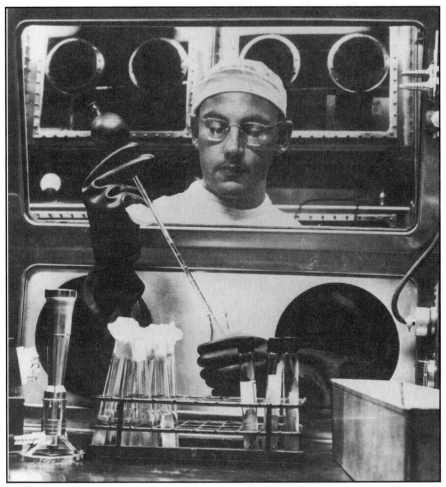

Using the "Glove Box" to handle highly infectious or dangerous materials.
US Army Photo

Many have requested information as to the qualifications of those selected. The medical qualifications for those participating does not enter the selection process. The thorough medical examination before they participate in medical experiments will be given after their arrival at the unit. The selection team looks for men with qualifications to do the various jobs in the unit. This would mean men able to train to operate intricate medical laboratory apparatus, men able to work with animals, men to work with statistics in offices, men to drive cars, men to work on medical wards, etc.

It must be stressed that the only connection the church has with this project is that the General Conference Committee studied the situation in 1954 when this program was set up and found that the program was one that a church member could feel free to participate in if he wished to do so. The decision to enter the project as a medical research volunteer must be the man's personal decision.

After selection to the unit the men will normally finish their medical AIT training at the Medical Training Center. Then they will be assigned to the unit at Fort Detrick, Frederick, Maryland. There they will be assigned duties as a medical soldier just as they would be assigned wherever they may serve. Since Fort Detrick is not able to provide work for all 175 men, some will be assigned to regular duty at Army medical installations nearby, such as Walter Reed Army Medical Center in Washington, D C. At some point during their active duty they will be given an opportunity to participate in a medical research program that will be carefully explained to them. This is still a volunteer program.

In the past there have been over 1,200 men who have participated in Project Whitecoat with no one having a medical problem extending beyond his duty time that has come as a result of his being in the program. This does not mean that the program is without danger. The whole program, however, is very carefully reviewed and checked by the outstanding civilian and military authorities in the field before any experimentation on human volunteers is undertaken.

Then on 7 July 1969, T. S. Geraty, Associate Secretary of the General Conference of Seventh-day Adventists, wrote a brief note as follows:

Elder R. H Pierson, President, Elder Theodore Carcich, Vice President, Elder N. C. Wilson, Vice President, Elder R. S. Watts, Vice President, Elder W J. Hackett, Vice President, Elder Theodore Lucas, YPMV Secy Elder Clark Smith, YPMV Assoc Secy Elder Charles Martin, YPMV Assoc Secy National Service Organization General Conference of SDA.

Dear Brethren:

REVIEW OF SDA PARTICIPATION IN "WHITECOATS"

In the light of the recent disclosures made public, such as Time essay, "The Dilemma of Chemical Warfare," in the June 27, 1969 issue of Time news magazine, page 20, it is essential in my considered judgment that the Seventh-day Adventist Church review its official encouragement and endorsement of Seventh-day Adventist servicemen participating unabashedly in the "Whitecoats Project."

With the issues of combatancy and noncombatancy, as conscientious cooperators and conscientious objectors we are vulnerable for duplicity and misunderstanding.

The General Conference officers responded to Doctor Geraty's suggestion by appointing a Whitecoat Study Committee composed of Neal C. Wilson, W.R. Beach, N.R. Dower, R.F. Waddell, M.D., T.S. Geraty, R.F. Osborn, W.H. Beaven, K.H. Wood, Stuart Nelson, M.D., Richard Hammill, and Clark Smith.

On 11 August 1969, the committee met. Members present were Neal C. Wilson, chairman, W.R. Beach, T.S. Geraty, C.D. Martin, Stuart Nelson, M.D., R.E. Osborn, J.R. Spangler, and K.H. Wood. The minutes of that meeting note:

BACKGROUND AND DISCUSSION

In the year 1954 Seventh-day Adventists were invited to participate in a program operated by the United States Army known as the United States Army Medical Research Institute of Infectious Diseases. This program, also known as Project Whitecoat, has been offered on a volunteer basis to all Seventh-day Adventists at Fort Sam Houston who have been through basic training or in the early weeks of Advanced Individual Training (AIT) until such time as their names are sent in for assignment. Up until August 1969, approximately 1500 Seventh-day Adventist young men have participated in this project.

In the discussion it was pointed out that in view of the recent interest shown in Project Whitecoat as well as the public attention given to chemical and biological warfare in general, it would be well to give a careful look at Project Whitecoat and all that is involved in the present program.

PLAN OF COMMITTEE ACTION

It was agreed that the following plan of committee action be followed:

1. *The National Service Organization will supply the members of the Project Whitecoat Study Committee with a list of questions which, from their back-ground and experience they feel should be answered concerning this project. The members of the study committee will suggest to the NSO any other questions which they feel should be included and then the NSO will compile a final list of questions concerning Seventh-day Adventist involvement in the White coat Project.*

2. *This final revised list will be placed in the hands of all committee members and also sent to the Commanding Officer of the Army unit, COL Daniel Crozier, MC. COL Crozier will be able to secure the necessary material from their file and make the preparation needed to answer questions raised.*

3. *The committee chairman will commission 4 or 5 committee members to go to Fort Detrick to see the facilities firsthand and discuss the questions with COL Crozier and his staff. Following the visit the delegation will make a report to the entire committee.*

4. *It was further felt that as soon as possible a written report should be presented to the church in general so as to clarify issues involved.*

Neal C. Wilson, Chairman
Charles Martin, Secretary Pro Tem

The appointed Whitecoat Study Committee was given the following Statements by Col. Crozier:

PROJECT WHITECOAT NOTES

The present name for this unit is the United States Army Medical Research Institute of Infectious Diseases.

This is an Army unit under Army control.

Seventh-day Adventists were chosen as a group to participate in this program for the following reasons:

1. *The group to be screened for volunteers must be large enough to produce the number of volunteers needed for the unit and small enough to be screened in a practical way.*

2. *Seventh-day Adventists are oriented toward medical service.*

3. *Seventh-day Adventist 1–A–Os in Basic and Advanced Individual Training at the Medical Training Center form a large enough unit to give the number of volunteers necessary and yet small enough to be a practical unit for the screening.*

4. *The usual procedure has been that any one who states that he is a Seventh-day Adventist is eligible. From the first day of arrival at the MTC, until they have progressed far enough into their AIT program so that names have been reported to Department of Army for assignment after AIT, are eligible.*

In October 1969, the General Conference officers investigated the proposed medical study unit and adopted the following statement:

STATEMENT OF ATTITUDE
REGARDING VOLUNTEERING FOR MEDICAL RESEARCH

August 1969 — To this time approximately 1500 Seventh-day Adventist young men have participated in the studies of Project Whitecoat. The procedure for volunteering for Project White coat is as follows:

1. *Twice a year (Spring and Fall) opportunity is given for volunteering for the project.*

2. *Since it is imperative that adequate information be given a volunteer before he will be accepted, the commanding officer of the United States Army Medical Research Institute of Infectious Diseases (Project Whitecoat) or his representative must interview the applicant.*

3. *Those accepted finish their Basic and Advanced Individual Training at the U.S. Army Medical Training Center and are sent to Fort Detrick, Maryland.*

4. *At Fort Detrick they are assigned duty with the Institute, or if there is no place for them to be assigned duty there, they are assigned to medical service duty at either Walter Reed Army Medical Center or Forest Glenn Annex.*

5. *If needed in a study, they are called and the entire study is explained to them. At this point they must again volunteer to participate.*

Doctor Geraty's query in July 1969 arose out of concerns expressed during his visits to Adventist academic institutions. Following the Study Committee's meeting in August 1969, he submitted several questions which he felt were pertinent to the Whitecoat study for presentation to USAMRIID:

In harmony with our suggested procedure and discussion of August 11, 1969, here are some questions relative to the "Project Whitecoat."

1. *Although the SDA Church ostensibly has the understanding that "These volunteers endanger their lives in time of peace in order to perfect means to combat disease in the Army and in the general population," is this the primary objective of the U.S. Armed Forces with "Project Whitecoat?"*

2. *Are the number of disciplinary problems among the volunteers discrediting the SDA Church? And do the U.S. Armed Forces recognize that not all volunteers are necessarily active church members?*

3. *Is "Church Preference" the category used in volunteer classification at the time of recruitment for "Project Whitecoat?"*

4. *Where is the line drawn in "Project Whitecoat" between defensive and offensive purposes for chemical and biological warfare?*

Ralph F. Waddell, M.D., Director of the world-wide health and medical programs of the Seventh-day Adventist Church suggested three questions, which were:

1. *How are individuals selected for the Whitecoat Project? Is such by personal election?*

2. *Upon completion of a term of duty with the Whitecoat Project, does the individual hold the same status as does a young man who has served his term of duty with the regular Military organization?*

3. *Are the research projects with which the Whitecoats are involved scientifically controlled, and are the results obtained of scientific value? Or is the entire project mainly a means of helping those who are noncombatants to fulfill their patriotic obligations according to the dictates of their consciences?*

On 4 September 1969, Clark Smith, Director, National Service Organization, mailed to Colonel Dan Crozier, MC, at Walter Reed Army Hospital, the proposed questions in anticipation of a conference on 11 September 1969. The following is a report of that conference:

REPORT OF PROJECT WHITECOAT
STUDY COMMITTEE

On Thursday afternoon, 11 September 1969, the group selected by Neal C. Wilson, Chairman of the Project Whitecoat Study Committee, visited Fort Detrick at Frederick, Maryland to present questions that had been gathered from the committee to the Commanding Officer of the U.S. Army unit known as Project Whitecoat.

The group consisted of W H. Beaven, President of Columbia Union College; Stuart Nelson, M.D., a practicing physician in Takoma Park; and the following General Conference personnel: T.S. Geraty, D.W. Hunter, J.C. Kozel, C.D. Martin, Philip S. Nelson, M.D., and Clark Smith.

COL Dan Crozier, USA, MC, Commanding Officer of Project Whitecoat, received the group cordially and answered factually the questions presented and any other questions asked by the group.

The questions and answers were as follows:

1. What is the official name for the unit known as "Project White-coat?"

A. *United States Army Medical Research Institute of Infectious Diseases (formerly known as the U.S. Army Medical Unit, Fort Detrick, Frederick, Maryland).*

2. How long has it been in existence?

A. *Established in 1956, but the basic concept was established in the 1953–54 period with the first project known as "CD-22" and carried on at Walter Reed Army Hospital.*

3.What is the official mission for the unit? What other objectives are there?

A. *Conducts studies related to medical defensive aspects of biological warfare and develops appropriate biological protective measures, diagnostic procedures and therapeutic methods.*

4. Can you furnish us with a bibliography of published reports that are the result of research work of this unit?

A. *Lists of Publications for the U.S. Army Medical Unit, Fort Detrick, Frederick, Maryland for the following dates: 1956–64, 1965, 1966, 1967, 1968 (in folder presented by Colonel Crozier; attached for committee members not on tour to Fort Detrick).*

5. Are the above reports generally available to the public?

A. *These reports are in such professional journals as:* Transactions of the Association of American Physicians, American Journal of Hygiene, Journal of Public Health, American Journal of Tropical Medicine and Hygiene, Armed Forces Epidemiological Board Medical Science Publications, Military Medicine Journal of Laboratory and Clinical Medicine, *as well as* Nature. *These were all gleaned from one page of the above Lists of Publications.*

A page-by-page examination of the journals indicates that all of them are freely available to the ethical investigator in any adequate medical library.

In addition, reprints of many of these articles are available to the ethical investigator in volumes bound by the year in which the articles were published. These reprints are also available in any adequate medical library. In short the reports are freely available.

6. *What non-military organizations benefit from the research done in this unit?*

A. *There have been 49 medical research institutions that have used experimental vaccines to protect their personnel engaged in research with infectious disease organisms. Benefits have also been extended internationally to such countries as Sweden, England and South America.*

7. *How does the unit fit into the organizational structure of the Defense Department? Is a profile or organization chart available?*

A. *The Commanding Officer of USAMRIID is directly responsible to the Commanding General of Medical Research and Development, who is directly responsible to the Army Surgeon General who is directly responsible to the Secretary of the Army. An organization chart is attached.*

8. *What connections are there between the defensive areas and offensive areas of research in the CBW field as carried an by the Defense Department?*

A. *The BW section USAMRIID is engaged in research in the defensive field. Its publications are freely available to all. Those working in the offensive field may utilize the information as any other interested party might do.*

The only other connection is that on rare occasions permission is requested for use by USAMRIID of a piece of experimental equipment costing in excess of a million dollars. Prudence on the part of the government does not allow both types of research to have identical items in this cost range.

9. Are the results of the research work carried on by this unit used directly or indirectly to improve bacteriological weapons of the U.S.?

A. Only in that the results as published could be picked up by other researchers and so used. This could be true of any published research by any unit.

10. How are protocols or study projects of the unit developed and actual study authorized? What controls outside the military can be exercised over the study projects?

A. In the study of an infectious disease when progress has been made to the point that it is necessary to get further information only by controlled exposure to the infectious organism, a request for such study in human volunteers is originated within the staff of USAMRIID. This request is studied and modified by the chiefs of each department. When they are satisfied that the request is justified and satisfactorily safeguarded as to protection of personnel in the study, the request is sent to the Commission of Epidemiological Survey of the Armed Forces Epidemiological Board. This group is composed of the leading infectious disease specialists in the United States. These men are heads of the department of medicine in leading medical schools and other areas.

The group studies the request and when satisfied that the information to be gained is necessary and can only be gained through the use of human volunteers and satisfied that the safeguards to volunteer personnel are adequate, they recommend to the Army Surgeon General that the studies be carried out. The Surgeon General has a separate group of specialists that go over the request to likewise satisfy themselves of the details. Then the Surgeon General recommends the request to the Secretary of the Army who has the request investigated to his satisfaction. Then the request is granted.

11. How does the volunteer subject know what is to be done to him personally? Does he know such things as:

> *—current status of the research?*
> *—approximate degree of danger he will be subjected to?*
> *—what safeguards are available to bring the study to an emergency conclusion?*

A. *The volunteer has the program in general explained to him at Fort Sam Houston at the time he volunteers for participation in the unit. After he arrives at Fort Detrick, when a project in which he will be asked to participate is coming up he will be a part of the group to which the entire matter is explained. This explanation will be done in both technical and lay terms. All questions by those in the group will be answered. Then the group will be interviewed individually so that any questions the volunteer might not have wanted to ask in the group can be answered. Then the volunteer will be asked to sign a consent statement.*

12. *How are the volunteer subjects screened and chosen?*

A. *Twice a year the Commanding Officer and another officer from USAMRIID go to the Army Medical Training Center at Fort Sam Houston, Texas. A member of the General Conference National Service Organization is also invited. Those 1–A–O classification men there who have stated their religious preference for the Seventh-day Adventist Church, who are in the Modified Basic Training or in the Advanced Individual Training (prior to the point where their names are submitted to Department of Army Headquarters for assignment orders after AIT) are brought together for an orientation. At this orientation the USAMRIID program is carefully explained and all questions concerning it are answered from the floor. The General Conference National Service Organization member states that the church feels that this is a humanitarian thing to do if there are those who wish to volunteer for the unit.*

Then the group is given an opportunity to consider the matter overnight. The next day each man is interviewed individually and any further questions are answered. Then he is given an opportunity to volunteer by signing the statement attached. From those signing this statement the officers from USAMRIID choose the number of volunteers needed.

13. *What volunteer subjects are used in the project other than those obtained from the Seventh-day Adventist 1–A–Os at Fort Sam Houston, Texas?*

A. *None*

14. *Are the number of disciplinary problems among the volunteers discrediting the SDA Church? Do the U.S. Armed Forces*

recognize that not all volunteers are necessarily active church members?

A. *Yes. The volunteers are chosen from those who have stated a religious preference for the SDA Church. No program of investigation as to the facts of personal standards or habits nor church membership is possible under the regulations of the U.S. Armed Forces. However, the Commanding Officer of USAMRIID pointed out that the disciplinary record of his unit has been so much better than the other two service units at Fort Detrick (or other military units) that he and his staff have been delighted with the personnel in the unit.*

Throughout the more than two hour interview members of the special group are encouraged to interrupt and ask any questions they had. At the conclusion each man was asked individually if he had any further questions. There were none.

A factor was pointed out by Colonel Crozier as significant. He indicated that not one project had been invalidated by actions of the participants.

The minutes of the next meeting of the Study Committee follow:

PROJECT WHITECOAT STUDY COMMITTEE
MINUTES

Thursday, 2 October 1969, 1 p.m., Room B

PRESENT Neal C. Wilson, chairman; W.R. Beach, W.H. Beaven, N.R. Dower, T.S. Geraty, D.W. Hunter, C.D. Martin, P.S. Nelson M.D., R.E. Osborn

PRAYER R.E. Osborn

REPORT: A report was presented by the group of men who had visited Fort Detrick on the 11th of September, giving the information obtained in the two hour interview, concerning Project Whitecoat, with COL Daniel Crozier, Commanding Officer of the Medical Research Unit. The group consisted of W.H. Beaven, T.S. Geraty, D.W. Hunter, J.C. Kozel, C.D. Martin, P.S. Nelson M.D., and Clark Smith. The report indicated a complete satisfaction with answers given by COL Crozier and an unanimous agreement with the program now being carried on.

SUGGESTED CHANGES AND ADDITIONS

As the entire Project Whitecoat Study Committee considered the report given, several suggested changes and additions were made. The revised report is being placed in the hands of all committee members.

COMMUNICATION TO THE FIELD

Next to be considered was the extent and method of communicating information concerning Project Whitecoat to the members in the churches. After considerable discussion, it was voted to recommend to the General Conference Officers the following:

1. That Kenneth H. Wood be asked to prepare an article for the Review & Herald — interview type was suggested — presenting the program as clearly and completely as possible, emphasizing the positive aspects of this humanitarian program. (This was published in the November 27, 1969 edition of the Seventh-day Adventist magazine "Review & Herald")

2. That Dr. W.H. Beaven be asked to write an article on Project Whitecoat to be sent to editors of the papers of all Seventh-day Adventist colleges and universities in the United States. (It was stated that Dr. Beaven had already written a letter to all presidents of the SDA colleges and universities in the United States presenting the favorable results of the committee's visit to Fort Detrick.)

Neal C. Wilson, Chairman
C.D. Martin, Secretary Pro Tem

Nevertheless, Doctor Beaven, in harmony with the above minutes, again wrote:

Columbia Union College
Takoma Park, Maryland
October 1969

TO: Editors, SDA College Newspapers

Dear Friends:

For the last several months questions have been raised in some quarters concerning Project Whitecoat carried on at the United States Army Medical Research Institute of Infectious Diseases at Fort Detrick, Frederick, Maryland. Some questions have been raised by Seymour Hersh in a book on chemical and biological warfare and in a subsequent article by him for the New York Times. The assertions have been made that Seventh-day Adventist young men have been engaged in studies directly related to the preparation by the United States for possible chemical/biological warfare.

Because these charges have been widely circulated, a committee entitled Whitecoat Study Committee was selected by the General Conference to investigate Project Whitecoat. On September 11, 1969, a sub-committee of the main committee visited Project Whitecoat at Fort Detrick, after having previously submitted an extensive list of questions to Colonel Dan Crozier, the commanding officer of the Project. There were eight members on this sub-committee, including two medical doctors, two educators, and representatives from the MV and other departments of the General Conference. I was a member of this committee. The report of this special group has been accepted by the Whitecoat Study Committee and has been submitted to the officers of the General Conference.

Because of the particular interest in this Project on Seventh-day Adventist college campuses, I am writing you for informational purposes only to give you a very brief summary of the results of this investigation. An extensive bibliography of findings was made to the sub-committee, and all questions raised by the committee were answered fully and frankly by Colonel Crozier to the satisfaction of the committee. At our October 2 meeting it was decided to recommend to the officers of the General Conference that an article embodying the major findings of this committee be subsequently published in the Review and Herald.

Project Whitecoat was established in 1956 at Fort Detrick for the purpose of conducting studies related to medical defensive aspects of biological warfare and developing appropriate biological protective measures, diagnostic procedures, and therapeutic methods. The Project has operated since that time, and since 1959 has been directed by

Colonel Dan Crozier. Research being conducted in Project Whitecoat is fully reported, and a bibliography of published reports is readily available. All of the reports are in Index Medicas. Further, there are publications and yearly compilations available in most medical libraries. Many of the studies are reported in the standard journals of the medical profession such as the Journal of Public Health, the American Journal of Tropical Medicine and Hygiene, and similar publications. All of these are freely available to the ethical investigator in any adequate medical library. In addition, the results of these studies are made available to other medical research institutions, and experimental vaccines have been used by them in the United States, Sweden, England, and countries of Central and South America. The research projects are thoroughly studied by boards of experts both within and without the armed services before they are undertaken and are fully monitored by these same experts during and after the research. None of the work of this organization is used directly or indirectly to improve bacteriological weapons of the United States.

The volunteers for the program are Seventh-day Adventists who are selected twice a year at Fort Sam Houston while undergoing training at the Army Medical Training Center. There are always many more volunteers than can be used; the number of men who have served in the unit at Fort Detrick in its total time is roughly 1500. Contrary to some popular reports, there is no evidence of permanent medical damage to any of the volunteers where definite results can be documented as having developed directly from Project Whitecoat activities. In one case the Army has honored a claim for a possible medical involvement since neither proof for or against the claim could be completely established. In every case for every project the man willingly volunteers to submit himself after having been thoroughly briefed.

Speaking personally now and not for the committee, I should like to say that I have lived in the Washington area since 1953, and in the ten years from 1959–1969 have been to Fort Detrick many times. The Project Whitecoat Unit is freely open for inspection; there are no locked or closed laboratories. If you have any reason to get on the post, you can visit everything that is related to Project Whitecoat. There is nothing classified, hidden, or secret. It is unfortunate, in my opinion, that the fully enclosed and classified medical unit that deals with chemical and biological warfare is immediately adjacent to the Project, and if there is any reason for using the material, I am sure it can be made available to you. You are free to use this letter in any way that *you see fit. If I can be of further service to you, I hope you will feel free to write.*

On 5 January 1970, the Secretary of the General Conference, Elder W.P. Bradley, wrote an interesting letter to Clark Smith in regards to a critic of the Church and Operation Whitecoat:

Dear Clark,

I have been interested in the correspondence which you have been sending to members of the NSO Committee about the inquiries of [a critic] regarding our part in the Whitecoat program.

I am not quite sure just what he is trying to prove in all of this and I am not sure whether his main thrust should be against the church or against the U.S. Army. I hope we don't become involved in defending the Army because of steps it takes to prepare itself for both offensive and defensive warfare. What good is any army if it doesn't take all precautions and make all preparations possible in order to be prepared for any contingency?

I understand our position with regard to military service is that we teach and advocate non-combatancy and we try to instruct our young men not to bear arms. On the other hand, however, we counsel them not to shrink from serving in the armed forces, to do their part faithfully and valiantly, and if one here and there decides to bear arms, we do not bring church discipline upon him for that.

I suppose some people would look upon a rifle as a defensive weapon and others would say it is offensive. The same thing can be of any type of warfare, including chemical and biological areas. If a young man drafted into the Army wants to choose to undergo this experimentation as a member of the Whitecoat group instead of going off to serve in Vietnam, I don't see why we shouldn't give him the privilege without being criticized for it. One thing I think we should be careful of and that is that we get ourselves into a position of defending the Army for everything it does in experimenting with and refining types of warfare which can be offensive as well as defensive. In other words, I don't think we ought to have to defend ourselves because the army engages in preparation for offensive warfare. If it is felt to that; in fact, I would like to ask him some questions about what his intentions are in all of this.

Given the strongly held views of separation of Church and State within the Seventh-day Adventist Church, it is not surprising there are those who are critical of the participation of church members in a medical research project run by the military. The controversy continues even today. There is no shortage of conspiracy theorists, and those with a political agenda, who view the Operation Whitecoat volunteers as stooges in a military (or CIA, DIA, or you pick the initials) scheme to develop the ultimate biological weapon. They prefer to ignore scientific facts which do not agree with their theories. They continue to be unpersuaded by truth and will likely remain so.

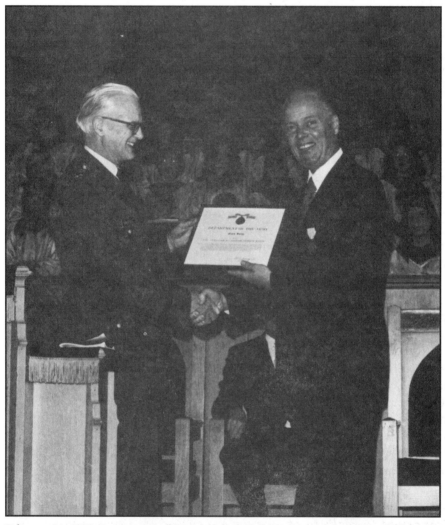

February 24, 1973. Presentation of Distinguished Civil Service medal to Elder Clark Smith, COL Dan Crozier, CDR, USAMRIID, Presenter.

REFLECTIONS OF WHITECOAT VOLUNTEERS

A unique feature in research utilizing humans is the ability to question them and share their reflections and emotional reactions, to ascertain why they were willing to take risks as subjects in medical research, and to learn their views regarding possible similar research involving their sons and/or daughters should future requests be made.

In order to achieve this goal, a simple questionnaire was prepared and mailed to all former Operation Whitecoat volunteers whose names and addresses were available. (The names of these individuals are listed later in this volume.) There were many whose names and addresses are unknown except in the recesses of military files now in permanent storage. It is believed, however, that the responses to the questionnaire are representative enough to provide a reasonably clear picture of the individuals and their reactions as recorded in 1991 and 1992, approximately twenty years after Operation Whitecoat ceased to function as a cohesive and designated medical research project.

Over two hundred responses to the questionnaire were received. These were coded with a number, but without additional identification in order to preserve anonymity of the former volunteers. Before examining the answers, it is well to remember that people tend to take certain courses of action for multiple reasons, some reasons being far more dominant or prominent than others. Some may be for obvious gain, some because it seems to be what others expect of you, some that are quite altruistic, and some because "it's the thing to do."

It must be remembered the men were draftees with limited personal choices of military assignment locations or military occupation or specialty coding; that during much of the time period covered by Operation Whitecoat the United States was involved in military conflicts in Asia and elsewhere; and that many Seventh-day Adventist pastors who served congregations where those men grew up had never been in the military so had little understanding of it. These pastors had a tendency to foster the belief that one must be a noncombatant if one were to be a "good" Seventh-day Adventist Church member. Thus the opportunity to help find answers to threatening diseases seemed an honorable way to serve both God and Country without moral or spiritual conflicts.

Records show that only about one in three of those who desired to volunteer for Operation Whitecoat could be accepted. It is important to realize not everyone accepted into such a large program would always meet the ideal standards of Adventism. The occasional failure or flaw of a given individual, while regrettable, did not flaw the concept or success of Operation Whitecoat anymore than the Judas issue defeated the purpose of the incarnation of Christ. In all wars or serious conflicts there are some casualties. In Vietnam, at Dien Bien Phu, General Giap, North Vietnam Commanding General, anticipated 100 percent casualties, yet won his battle and drove the French from Vietnam.

Analysis of Answers to the Questionnaire

Question pertaining to educational level

It seems obvious that the educational levels of the Whitecoat volunteers were sufficiently high that they would not blindly react and volunteer without some meaningful rationale. From tabulation of the 201 answers returned, the educational levels at the time of Whitecoat involvement and compared to 1991–1992 were:

	Then	Now
No answer	4	4
Grade 8	1	1
Grade 9	1	1
Grade 12	60	41
Grade 13	48	12
Grade 14	29	16
Grade 15	10	4
Bachelor's Degree	55	67
Master's Degree	3	36
DDS	0	5
MD	0	7
PhD	0	6
Dmin	0	1
Total	201	201

One of this volume's writers (RLM) served as chaplain at two Navy Basic Training Centers during the draft era, and recalls that the educational level of the draftees was higher than enlistees prior to the draft, but was not as high as these volunteers'. Their subsequent educational levels reveal continued educational achievement. As many volunteers noted, Operation Whitecoat gave them an opportunity to see the educational possibilities and privileges before them. For some, military service provided the additional financial resources needed to pursue educational and professional goals. In addition, work assignments within Operation Whitecoat provided self discipline and motivation for greater achievement.

It is important to keep the educational levels and age factors in mind as the questionnaire answers are examined and evaluated. Adventists are generally upwardly mobile and above average in educational achievements. This is due in part to a vibrant Church-sponsored educational system as well as to a sense of individual responsibility.

Questions pertaining to age

The questionnaire requested the date of birth and the date of beginning military service as a draftee (1–A–O) and on to Project Whitecoat. Two hundred sixteen questionnaires were tabulated, with the following results:

Age	Number
18	10
19	18
20	30
21	38
22	37
23	46
24	19
25	7
26	2
27	1

If the educational levels and age groupings are projected for the full number of 3,000 Operation Whitecoat volunteers, it would not be difficult to understand how these men as a homogeneous group made an excellent resource for the various medical and vaccine testing programs. These factors, combined with similar life-style beliefs and practices, tended to make experimental findings more accurate than if a more heterogeneous group of men had been utilized.

Question pertaining to SDA Church membership

The questionnaire asked the age at which the individual volunteers became members of the Adventist Church through the ritual of baptism by immersion, which is considered the doorway into the Church. Two hundred nine individuals responded giving their baptismal ages as:

Age	Number
9	4
10	18
11	16
12	80
13	25
14	25
15	8
16	9
17	3
18	4
19	0
20	4
21	3
22	1
2	32

These ages imply that a large percentage of the Whitecoat volunteers were raised in homes that were friendly to Adventism, were adherents or were members of the Church. Thus the stance of the Church as generally perceived by many pastors and members would have significant influence in the choices made for military service when some freedom of choosing was possible.

Questions pertaining to marital status

Of the 209 individuals who answered the question, "Were you married when you became a Whitecoat volunteer?," 80 said they were married at that time, 38.3 percent of the total respondents.

To the question, "Are you married to the same individual?," 55 of the married respondents (68.8 percent) said Yes. Of the 25 who said they were not married to the same individual (31.3 percent), 23 were divorced (28.8 percent) and the remaining two had lost their marriage partners by death (2.5 percent).

None of the 80 men who were married when they began Operation Whitecoat believed that the Whitecoat experience had a negative effect on their marriages. In contrast, some readily admitted that they were willing to be medical experimental volunteers in order to avoid probable separations due to military orders.

Question: Do you know of any residual effects of Operation Whitecoat on your health? If so, what are these?

To date, only one Operation Whitecoat participant has been awarded a service connected disability—at 80 percent because there are no absolute certainties with regard to the cause of the disability. The government awarded the disability rather than continue a court battle with an uncertain outcome. A few other Whitecoat participants believe their current medical problems are Whitecoat related, but reviews of their charts, as well as medical examinations, have not confirmed this view. USAMRIID still expresses a willingness to review any records and do medical work-ups on any participant who presents sufficient medical evidence to indicate need of follow-up attention. Some cases were forwarded to USAMRIID as a result of research for this volume.

It is acknowledged that in chemical research done prior to the official start of Operation Whitecoat the Army Chemical Service did some experiments that may have created problems for some participants. The Whitecoat project, by contrast, was purely a medical research program. Unfortunately, the media sometimes either did not understand the separation of chemical research from that of medical research or on some occasions deliberately mixed them in support of a hidden agenda. Evidence supporting this statement is in the archives of both the Army and the Seventh-day Adventist Church's General Conference offices. (In like manner, the questionnaires being discussed are in the General Conference archives for possible future research efforts.)

A few respondents indicated that they believe their eyesight problems, heart ailments, impotency, muscular weaknesses, or mental status may be residual effects of Whitecoat experiments. A study of their particular Whitecoat experimental research project has not provided any clear evidence connecting these issues. Moreover, within such a large group of individuals it would be unusual if over the period of 40 years a number of medical problems should not be manifested. Even the Army cannot always conquer genetic factors nor combat exposure to illness-causing circumstances in human life.

It may well be that in peace time, when no obvious international conflict requires American military presence, parents may not favor their sons or daughters being involved in potentially life-threatening research. But when body-bags begin arriving back in America, the choice of a controlled environment with the best medical skills available may not seem quite as dangerous as the battlefield. When such conditions exist, it is not just an academic discussion; rather it is perceived as a life and death dilemma.

Some of the respondents who expressed negative feelings with regard to their children's possible participation in future medical research, indicated unhappiness that they were not given the findings of the experiments directly, promptly and individually. While this may well be true, it needs to be remembered that the scientific mind groping for exact answers to difficult questions may not necessarily place patient relations at the forefront. Moreover, many such experiments require extended time periods for data to be correlated, results finalized and prepared for release. Added to these factors is that of the military environment where orders or assigned tasks are to be executed without a full explanation of the "Whys" or expectations on final results. Thus while the Commanding Officers are repeatedly praised by the Whitecoats, the system did not and does not promote a sense of personal identity and recognition for achievements, but for exceptional instances.

Can you list some of the reasons you chose to participate in Operation Whitecoat?

As mentioned earlier, human decisions are usually made for multiple reasons with one or more of them seemingly more prominent. This is borne out by the respondents' answers. The remarkable feature of the responses is their patent frankness and honesty. Even when the answer seemed so obviously self serving, they were quite candid. This was true even when they signed their names, as they all did.

Fifty of the 209 responses to this question gave avoiding duty in Korea or Vietnam as one of their reasons for volunteering as a Whitecoat participant. These men did not run to Canada nor use influence to avoid the draft; rather, when given the option to be human volunteers in scientific studies against virus or germs, they chose the course that seemed best to them under their circumstances. Among the factors considered by these volunteers were the following: Some were newly married (80 of the 209); some were expecting a baby shortly; some 15.8 percent were influenced by family pressure and their own fears. Some 13.9 percent volunteered because of Church support, either through direct promotion of the project or by their own beliefs and training as conscientious objectors in the Church's Medical Cadet Corps. Forty-seven of the respondents indicated that they volunteered for Whitecoat in order to assist in finding answers to reduce human pain and misery in harmony with the Church's teachings.

Other reasons included:

—Desire to stay stateside, close to home.

—Cross-train professionally in medical skills.

—Learn more microbiology, as it was my chosen profession.

—Considered it a worthwhile medical research project.

—The openness and apparent fairness of Whitecoat briefers was impressive.

—The privilege of choosing one's own duty in the impersonal military system.

—The ability to continue profession as a medical illustrator.

—The opportunity to be in an Adventist atmosphere even in the Army.

—The glamour that Whitecoat seemed to offer.

—An excellent way to serve one's country and remain in America at the same time.

—The privilege of contributing to health care long after military duties completed.

The various answers are reflective of many factors. Having been raised in the aftermath of World War II and with an awareness of the terrible effects of any war, it would be natural to wish to avoid armed conflict insofar as possible. When the number of casualties among the ranks of corpsmen and medics of World War II is recalled, there was reason enough for the sensible to consider possible arenas of service that would not violate their understanding of Church teachings regarding "Thou shalt not commit murder." Having been exposed in schooling and Church to the examples of the great medical scientists held up as heroes, some saw in Whitecoat the opportunity to also make significant contributions to the healing of mankind. And they did!

> *The questionnaire concluded by saying, "Please use the bottom of this page and the back of this questionnaire for any additional comments you care to make; add as many additional sheets as needed. Inasmuch as this is a research project involving veterans, please use the enclosed pre-addressed and franked envelope for your answers."*

It is significant that a good number of former Whitecoat participants took the time and effort to reflect and write of their experiences and reactions. Perhaps their comments are the best guide to their Whitecoat experience as they look backward at what their participation accomplished. In keeping with the promise not to identify individuals without their prior consent, all answers are coded. The responses are given with little editing or intervening comments in order that they may tell their stories.

Some Answers to the Questionnaire

#7. The Major and Colonel I worked with were very caring people. They were a pleasure to work with from day to day and professional in relations You wanted to be a part of the team because of their spirit, not because of fear for some command being barked out.

I'll not soon forget a Col. when an "in-project" started once. The patients weren't getting sick like they were suppose to. As I remember, they were an hour or two past due to be sick. He was pouring over data with concern he'd done some-

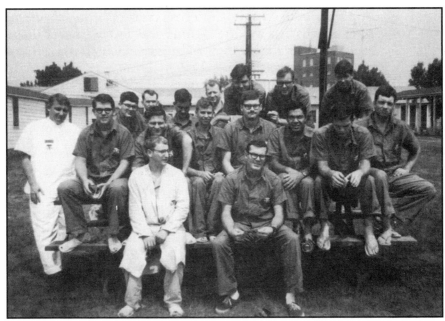

Rift Valley Fever project volunteers take an outdoor break from hospital routines

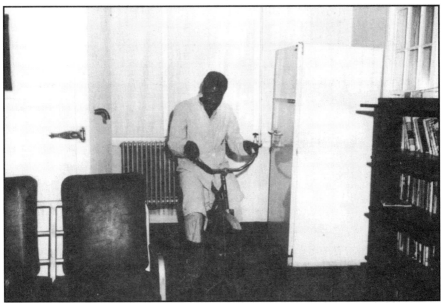

Keeping fit calls for creativity when you are confined to the hospital. The stationary bike helps provide an opportunity.

thing wrong. To watch the stress slacken as the last of the patients got ill, gave me a glimpse of the pressures these research people were really under. To watch them function gave me confidence.

It was my understanding that when Whitecoats got press, that the Col. would answer to the Pentagon concerning details. I never did see his rebuttal in print in those National papers.

#11. I can say that my experience in Operation Whitecoat was very rewarding. Besides working with other Christians we also worked with some great staff. I am [indebted] to one Dr. for her training and personal interest in our lives. I really learned Bacteriology from her. I could say that my experience in her department motivated me to focus my education in Microbiology, Medical Technology and Public Health. Ft. Detrick was a launching pad for me. Since graduating from college, I have been involved in establishing a school of Medical Technology, two Health Sciences Departments, a four year college in Virginia and now a school of Public Health here at the University of Montemorelos, in northeastern Mexico.

I would also like to pay tribute to a Colonel who showed great interest to the fellows in or out of projects. I still remember seeing him standing in the light of the doorway early AM after I had gotten out of the heat chamber. My head felt like a sledgehammer was beating away on the inside. Needless to say I wasn't getting to sleep very quickly. His kind attention to our needs really impressed me.

#22. In the late fall of 1963 or early spring 1964 I was involved in a strange incident. I was assigned as a Corpsman on ward 200 at Detrick. A civilian technician came in who had been involved in a spill behind the fence. They weren't sure exactly what he had been exposed to. He complained of high fever, headaches and various pain. He was admitted and I was one of several Corpsmen assigned to take care of him. After about 2 days his condition got worse and he was placed in isolation. I was again one of the Corpsman assigned to his room. This required that we spent the better part of our 8 hr. shift in cap, masks and gown in his room. It was about this time that they decided he had been exposed to Bolivian Hemperadiac [sic] Fever. We were told that this could be a very fatal disease. Within 7 days the man died. After his death, all of us who had been exposed to him were given the option of getting a shot of a vaccine which I understood was experimental and had been developed at Boston Medical Center. There was enough serum as I remember for 12 people only. So we had a list based on those who had the highest amount of exposure. If anyone didn't want the shot then it was available to someone else further down the list. As I recall the first 12, including me, took the shot. I've never heard that there were any side effects.

One of the projects that was most interesting was the heat project where they make you sick, cured you, then put you in a hot room for 24 hours to collect sweat. The room temperature was as high as 114 degrees F; humidity was close to 100 percent. I didn't serve on one of those projects but I was a Corpsman on one.

#23. Participation in Operation Whitecoat was a unique experience for me... I met some very fine people and had occasion to travel a bit.

The staff treated us well and were very considerate of our needs. During my 8 week confinement at Fort Detrick the staff did everything possible to make us comfortable and happy. I received expert and excellent medical care during my illness and subsequent recuperation. At no time did I ever entertain any thoughts of danger or adverse effects to my health.

#28. If you are interested in the overall aspects of my experience, here are my comments! The overall experience was pleasurable. I enjoyed the scientific aspects of radiation monitoring I learned in my military job and took pride in organizing the film badge department.

When on project, I enjoyed the camaraderie and liked helping the others, when I was well and they were ill. I would love to know the reason I either did not get sick (2 projects) or showed resistance for a time (1 project).

#39. I know of an interesting situation that occurred. There was a soldier in my basic training class who was not an SDA. After basic he was a part time company clerk during our medic training. When the orders came back to all the soldiers selected for the Whitecoats, the clerk typed his name on the orders. This clerk went to Washington, DC like the rest of us SDAs. He was an attorney before being drafted, and we became good friends during our stay in Washington. I don't believe that anyone ever found out that he wasn't an SDA or that he never interviewed for the Whitecoats.

#48. I hope positive things come from this endeavor because humanly speaking this will give some individuals an out to voice their disapproval for the project.

#56. I think a section of your book should be on the social existence of community Whitecoat families. Also the very important role of the Frederick Church in supporting us over the years.

#58. Overall, I enjoyed the Whitecoat Project. I felt that we as a group were treated very nicely and I don't have any complaints. I look back at the 18 months that I spent at Walter Reed as good ones with pleasant memories.

#61. I never was involved in a project from a "guinea pig" basis, but I did work in serology as a lab assistant. We became good friends and I even visited on several occasions. Because of my wife's illness and eventual death while in the service, I was not asked to participate in a project myself. After the death of my wife the men on the base "passed the hat" and this covered a large portion of the funeral expenses. I was very much appreciative of and touched by their concern in my hour of need. I had a 9 month old son at the time. That same son is now attending Columbia Union College in Takoma Park, Md. I look back on my years as a "Whitecoat" with good memories and if the opportunity came my way again, I would not be afraid to do my part.

#68. When I worked there, our work was classified. We didn't even talk to each other about what we did. We were programmed not to talk. To this day I find it against the grain to talk about what we did, so I have never talked about it. There really wasn't much to talk about.

It is going to be interesting to see what people come up with. It wasn't a heroic job—just a job. I fail to see the reason for a book. Is someone or organization wanting to gain favor? I'm for the reunion and even the book. I just wonder why?

#75. I worked in maintenance and fabrication in the old 1412 building. We built whatever was needed for the research projects and general building maintenance. I did not participate in any of the projects.

#79. Participation in Whitecoat was no hardship to me. I lived off post. It was essentially an 8:00 to 5:00 job. My selection into Whitecoat was, in my mind a miracle. Space does not allow a full telling but I was selected without an interview and while on my 8th week of AIT. I can supply further details if necessary. I'm glad someone is putting together a history of Whitecoats. I feel that it is an important undertaking.

#84. As I recall in the project I was on, everyone except one person was well by the end of the project. That one person stayed 3 or 4 days then was released. On another project I heard about men were required to work out mathematical problems even while sick with a fever. On this project men got very sick. Some even had intravenous injections, but in time all recovered. They got far sicker than planners expected.

On another project participants had blood drawn every hour around the clock for 3 days except between 3:00AM and 6:00AM when they could sleep uninterrupted.

On all projects where blood was drawn men were paid $25.00 for a pint (or more) if more blood drawn at end of project. They were also given extra leave time (in addition to regular leave granted each year). Most men seemed to feel projects were well screened and safely conducted, and there were always enough volunteers for the projects. We were not told the results of the experiments though. No follow up 6 months or 1 year later.

#87. During my final months I became very ill with what was described as "some kind of encephalitis" by the physicians at Detrick. I spent a week in the hospital. The problem has reoccurred over the years. I would like my medical records for that time.

#97. In the 23 years since I left Fort Detrick I have used and built on all the skills I learned in the Army laboratory. First, I did a medical technology internship and obtained my Registry as an MT (ASCP) in the clinical lab. All those days of doing the calculation for statistical analysis paid off in moving rapidly into supervision, quality control and eventually computer hardware and software engineering and programming. I finished 15 years in lab work as Chief Medical Technologist of a commercial clinical lab without reaching the limit of the microbiology, chemistry or hematology and virology pioneered there, but only very recently!

I have no regrets or knowledge of harm to anyone. I am thankful to the NSO, and the Frederick SDA congregation for their support and caring love.

#107. To me the Whitecoats was just a job, and a simple job at that. Most of the men I knew, including myself, wanted to go on project simply because we got a few days off and a few extra dollars. Looking back on it, that was a most foolish reason, but considering our age we believed most of what we were told—that being, everything was perfectly good. To date I have not heard of anyone who suffered any lasting ill effects of the Whitecoat Project. The time I was in, Nov. '71 to Sept. '73, only 2 or possibly 3 projects occurred using humans.

#120. I believe Project Whitecoat was a useful experience for me. Developing discipline and following through on work projects has been a benefit for me in my work experience.

#129. I felt at the time and still believe my welfare was kept paramount during the experiment in which I participated. Indeed, I and others felt some guilt at how we lived when other SDAs were dying in Vietnam.

Fort Detrick was frightening, however. I knew about the LSD experiments and I routinely went into the Hot Area and heard stories about fatalities (true?). So I was aware that some terrible business was being conducted there while I put airplane models together and watched movies.

#134. I felt very fortunate to get into the Whitecoats. I look back now and realize I was probably very trusting as I did not think of the possible problems that I might have had. However, when viewed from the perspective of total danger to Army personnel it posed no additional threat. I was very fortunate as I received no disease. I believe God was looking out for me as He always has. Good luck in your research.

#147. I joined the Army after 8 months being out of college. I was a science major. I was told that I would work in the science lab at Whitecoat. But what bothered me is that I got to do things that any high school freshman could do while guys who were English and philosophy majors got to assist with the real experiments. (But I suppose that was typical Army then.) I appreciate the Army providing the kinds of food we as SDAs could eat. Not so during basic, even at Fort Sam.

I appreciated the support of the Frederick Church. I was a black soldier in a white world. Although I could not date any of the white girls, I was made to feel welcome at the Church and its functions. Most of the black guys went to D.C. for social outlet. I did not like to have to rush to D.C. at other people's convenience just to see girls. So staying on base and going to the Frederick Church was a blessing even though they had no black girls.

#149. My tour of duty in the Army was about as good as a soldier could ask for due to becoming accepted into the "Project Whitecoat!" I was a college graduate, with a B.A. degree in Business Admin., from Pacific Union College, and was selected by the Whitecoat C.O. at the time to become his new Supply Sergeant for the Company, but I had already rented an apartment in the Takoma Park area, so I was assigned to the Microbiology Lab - subsection from Fort Detrick. It was located at the Kelser section (animal compound) which was also a subsection of Forrest Glen. I was then assigned to work as a lab assistant in the Biochemistry section of that building. The whole Microbiology building I was working in, as my duty assignment, was dedicated entirely to the study, etc., of Bubonic Plague. I was therefore vaccinated for the Plague and had to wait 2 weeks before being allowed into the "working" area of the building, since it was considered a "HOT" Lab. I worked, hands on, with the live virus (Pasteurella pestis) performing various biochemistry testing in the isolation of molecular sizes of the Plague virus protein. When I ended my tour of duty I was tested for my blood "Titer" against Bubonic Plague so records could be updated. Anyhow, I was told by the Commanding Officer of the Lab, that my blood "Titer" for plague was the highest of any recorded to date (that was the summer - August of 1970). I thought this scenario might be of some interest/importance for Whitecoat records.

#150. I am very glad I had the opportunity to participate in Operation Whitecoat. I met many wonderful friends and I felt that I was serving my country in a meaningful way. The Project gave me a chance to come to Washington, D.C. where I met my wife of 25 years. So, I have a wonderful wife and 2 lovely children, thanks to Operation Whitecoat.

#151. I am amazed that the Frederick Church is now interested in Whitecoats. When I was stationed there and Linda and Bob talked me into going to Church I felt anything but welcome. The preacher there made reference from the pulpit to my "costume"—in Oklahoma my jacket, hat and cowboy boots were not out of place as dress at Church or camp meeting. I was stunned, embarrassed and determined never to go back.

Sarge at bldg. 1040, and Bill (civilian) went way beyond call of duty in their help and guidance of many of us who worked there.

#152. I have had some health problems but I don't know if they are related to Q Fever. I didn't show any symptoms at the time of the experiment. I would be interested in knowing what the experience of others has been who were involved in the Q Fever Project.

#153. I volunteered for the Whitecoat Project in May '71 and did so mainly to stay out of Viet Nam. Even though the war was winding down they still had a shortage of medics and many that were graduating were still going. The day that I was selected there were approximately 250 GIs in the auditorium who all wanted one of the only 56 slots for Project Whitecoat.

Other than being SDA they were looking for men who had other civilian training that could be useful. So just being SDA did not always mean you were automatically chosen. (A guy I grew up with was at the auditorium where recruits were being selected. He was SDA also but did not get chosen. I was pretty homesick at the time and he had seen me stand to ask a question about Project Whitecoat. Neither of us knew the other was in the service but after the meeting he ran up to me and gave me a big hug. I never saw him after that and still don't know what became of him.) I was a registered x-ray tech when I was drafted and they had a million volt x-ray machine that they used to irradiate the animals that they gave certain diseases to see if they could kill the disease before

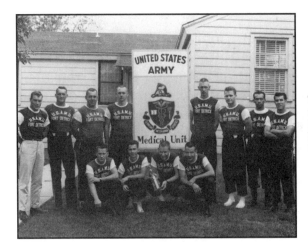

The medical unit teams were frequent winners at Ft. Detrick. Ballgames helped break the routine for many Whitecoats.

For those who were confined to the wards there were indoor recreation options...

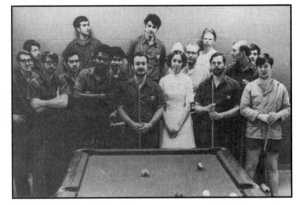

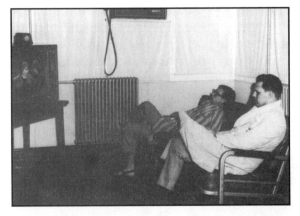

...including the ever popular "I Love Lucy" on the good old black & white T.V.

killing the animal. So they chose me. As it ended up, however, after I arrived at Fort Detrick they needed a x-ray tech in the dispensary and that's where I ended up working.

Other than short episodes of pure terror, most of the time it was just like any other job. The terror part came ever so often when one of the scientists upstairs broke vials and contaminated themselves with a deadly disease that at that time had no cure and generally ended in the death of the person involved. And more than once I had to put on special isolation garb to go in and take a chest x-ray under the watchful eyes - outside of the isolation lab of course - of high ranking officers to see if I broke the isolation. If you did, then you weren't allowed out. The disease was Ky Co Mungo [sic] disease, from South America. I wore double gloves booties, gowns and scrubs plus a special helmet that filtered the air I breathed. Coming out I had to shower twice and stand under ultra violet light.

Living in the barracks had its surprises too. Although a lot of SDAs were involved in Project Whitecoat, we were just a small number of the men on the base. And though being raised as SDA didn't change the fact that things of the world weren't before us at times. As I found out one Sunday morning on my way to the shower, there were a lot of guys lined up outside of one of the bays where a prostitute was working. Right there in the barracks!! How she got on a secure base I never found out. However, sick call was up after she left.

As with a lot of things there comes a time when you have to pay up and Project time was that time. Though I only participated in one project, at the time that was one too many. I was never the hero type and even after they explained to me what to expect I wasn't convinced. There just seemed something wrong with injecting something in me that was going to make me sick. The yellow fever and encephalitis project was what they called an outpatient project. That meant that you didn't have to be isolated from the public. Prior to the injection you were briefed as to what to expect. We were told that approxi-

mately 24 hours following the injection we would become feverish, have joint pain and our skin would feel as
though it had gotten a bad sunburn. In fact when it hit me
my wife and I were at the shopping center right outside of
the base and she had to drive us back home. I could
hardly bend my arms and knees to get out of the car when
we got home and my wife had to help me in the house.
Here I was 22 years old and I walked like I was 80. I was
lucky though, because I got better in about 2 days. One of
my closest friends had to be admitted to the ward for 2
weeks because he became so ill.

I look back at that time in my life and ask if I would ever
volunteer for something like that again. And I would
have to say that I really don't know. At the time most believed that the U.S. was involved in an unjust war. Dem-
onstrators were outside of the gates protesting the
supposedly biological bombs we were secretly making.
And the President of the U.S. was asking the public to forget something called Watergate and focus on what he
was doing to end the Viet Nam war. I think that if these
were different circumstances and felt that I could trust
my government, knew what I was doing was solely to
help and not hurt, I would do it again.

As I'm sure other SDAs were, I was proud of the uniform
I was wearing. And looking back at that time, it feels good
to know that at a time when so much bad was happening,
that just maybe I was doing something good.

#156. I enjoyed Whitecoat very much. The atmosphere to work,
to grow up, the historical eastern seaboard, and the Nation's Capital. I was able to meet people from all over the
world and come across these people from time to time and
even meet others who were there before me. I received an
education about people I could never have learned in a
classroom setting. I grew up in two years and am better
prepared to function and produce in this world.

I enjoyed the freedom of athletics the Army offered softball football, tennis, and golf.

Working around a lab and somewhat involved with the medical area I learned much that has helped me to work in a public hospital and be prepared for various events. I learned to keep my head in emergencies and to help others as best as I can in stressful situations. And the GI Bill which the Government provided helped me to receive 3 years of college and 2½ of graduate school. Living outside of the USA now makes me think more of how good we have it there. I am able to see some good and some bad and know that America is a great place.

#163. Being raised in Arkansas, "Rabbit Fever" or Tularemia was a feared sickness when I was a kid. I have always wondered if the vaccination was good and if it was of value to the good of medical progress.

I and some of my friends were not good SDAs and there was a movement to have us disfellowshipped. But some were in our favor-we, like all sinners, had no defense. But some fellow GIs came to our defense. I would like to thank them someday.

I could go on and on, but won't bore you. Thanks for your efforts and may God Bless them. I hope He comes though before you finish and we can all discuss these things face to face in Heaven.

#167. I'm enclosing some thoughts and recollections of my days in "Whitecoats" ('65 –'67). I was on two projects in '66—one, a 3-day "Cold Project," and an August '66 week "Tularemia" Project. I've had no negative effects over the years to my knowledge.

Best of luck on the book. I've felt a book has long needed to be written. I remember in the late 70's when the projects were declassified. Within one day a Dayton reporter had my name and contacted me. People seem to automatically think of the worst when you say you were a "Human Guinea Pig."

#168. California Rabbit Fever (4 weeks duration): We were placed in the hospital ward for 2 weeks prior to being injected with the virus. (Six of us, including myself, were controls, and the other six were injected.) During the 4 weeks of the project, we were given measured amounts of fruits, charcoal, and other foods to eat. We were also required to drink a prescribed amount (½ or 1 gal.) of an oily liquid drink mix each day.

The six that were injected at the end of the 1st 2 weeks got really sick with nausea, vomiting, aches, cramps, etc. The other six of us just continued along as normal. Blood, stool samples, weights, temps, etc. were taken daily. We were allowed to paint pictures, build models, read, play cards, etc., but not to exercise, or be outside for any length of time.

One man got so sick, that even on his leave time after the project, he was re-admitted to a hospital in Indianapolis, IN and spent much of his 4 weeks leave there.

Metabolism and Heat Chamber Project (2 weeks duration). We were admitted to ward 603 of US Army on 17 July 1963 and were kept there for 2 weeks. Weights, temperatures, blood pressures, etc., were taken frequently, but otherwise we were not required to do much during that time. We were placed in the heat chamber for a period of 24 hours. Steam was injected into the chamber until the room temperature was 104 and our bodies slowly increased until they were also at that temperature. We were required to drink 8 oz. glass of warm water every ½ hour to keep our sweat loss to a minimum. We were hooked up to various instruments (temp, etc.) and asked to perform various tasks during those hours. The Doctors were changed every ½ to 1 hour so as not to be affected by the temperature. I can only remember the first 6 hours or so in the chamber because of my heat-caused delirium. Another of the volunteers started kicking, screaming and trying to climb the walls, so they removed him from the chamber early. They told me later that I had tried to leave the chamber to "get my robe," but I have no recollection of that event. My next memory was being helped up the hallway of the building to my room (at the end of the 24 hour test).

#174. Until I was drafted, I had never been east of Nevada, and had never flown in an airplane. My Army experience helped me learn about my country and its people. I appreciated the servicemen's centers in San Antonio, Washington D.C. and Frederick. It was at Frederick that I was first elected as a Church Deacon.

Our being 300 miles away from our parents brought us closer together as a family. I wish we could have kept that closeness.

#197. My total involvement in Whitecoat lasted 10 days. I did think it was unusual that I was always picked to drive a carload of Whitecoats to Ft. Detrick when I was a control. This was for the monthly follow-ups.

Nobody at Ft. Sam Houston ever verbally told me when I was picked for Whitecoat. I found out from a list taped to a Church door. I will be pleased to help in your project in any way since I thought Whitecoat was forgotten and it came at the high point in my personal life too.

#204. A specific medical problem was discovered that would not have been found if I had remained in the Army other than in "Whitecoats."

RECOLLECTIONS OF OPERATION WHITECOAT

Merlin D. Bitzer

I am writing this long overdue letter to you since I had promised Chaplain Mole I would get the following information to him long before he passed away. However, due to my usual procrastination, I have delayed it until now.

Chaplain Mole was interested in the following information for his book because of my work with the Whitecoat Projects and my continued military Career.

Both my brother and I were subjects for the projects. My brother, Llewellyn (Lou) Bitzer was a subject in just one of the studies and he has not kept in touch with you at all. I will enclose his address in this letter. He was at Walter Reed from 1962–1964.

I was stationed at Walter Reed and Ft. Detrick from 1962 until 1965 and worked in the labs for COL William Biesel on the specimen collection and analysis of them on the first Auto analyzer equipment in the medical research lab. During that time I also was a subject in 3 studies, one [of which was a] metabolic[ally] balanced study, which meant we were on the diet of soybean milk and fruit for a 28 day period. Half way through this study we were infected with tularemia via aerosol masks in a gas chamber like unit and, of course, monitored closely. The second study was one in which the researchers wanted to find out if we could be re-infected with tularemia and we spent 21 plus/minus days in the unit, but were fed a regular diet and treated according to the degree of our infection. The third study I participated in was the hyperthermic study in which we again placed on the metabolic[ally] balanced diet. After a good base line was obtained, we were taken into a heated room where our body temperature was raised to 103 degrees over an 18 hour period and then held there for 6 hours.

Because I had participated in the 2 studies in which tularemia was used, Dr. Biesel asked me if I would be able to participate in this third study. The reason being, he felt he could gather valuable data from a volunteer that had gone through all three projects. He also felt that it was easier for me to be a subject in a third project since I worked with them on an ongoing basis.

I had extended in the Army for an 11 month period at Fort Detrick and was discharged in January of 1965. I rested in March of 1965 and went to Germany where I served in the 8th Field Evacuation Hospital until January of 1968.

After being discharged from the Army in 1968, I began working as home health aid caring for the super wealthy in the north side of Chicago and started night school at a junior college. 1969 found me beginning my formal nursing education at Andrews University, which I completed in June of 1973 with my Major in nursing and a minor in behavioral science, giving me my B.S. in nursing.

I was commissioned in the U.S. Navy in November of 1973 and served until 31 December, 1988 as a Nurse Corps Officer...I retired at the rank of Lieutenant Commander.

It was my understanding that of the 5000 [Sic] Whitecoat volunteers, I was the only one that ended up finishing a 21 year military career and retired as a Commissioned Officer. This of course was another point of interest that Chaplain Mole had wanted to discuss. The reason that I had done this was because I had been a kid with little sense of direction and little to no self esteem. My enlisted time helped me achieve both of these through the schools the Army sent me to. The most important one being the Non-Commissioned Officers Academy in Bad Tolez, Germany. After that experience, I had the necessary self-confidence to get a college education.

18 March 1998

Sorry for not getting this information to you sooner, but I will try to finish this letter today. As you will note, I started this letter in 1996 and have not finished it as I doubted it would be of any value at that late date. Just a few closing lines and I will get the letter in the mail.

During the 15 years I spent as an officer in the Navy, I completed my master's [degree] in business in 1983. In September, 1981 I was diagnosed with histiocytic lymphoma and treated at Naval Regional Medical Center, San Diego. Besides the chemotherapy, I was fortunate enough to have a physician who attended our church and who was at the time working with the Livingston Clinic, an alternate therapy clinic owned and then operated by two Adventist doctors, Dr. Livingston and Dr. Wheeler. [They] gave me some instruction in the use of Megavitamin therapy both orally and IV, which I followed at home. Interestingly enough, of 4 people that I knew about with the same disease at the time I had it and was getting chemo and they were also. I was the only one of the group to add the alternative therapy and I was the only one to survive.

I had called Colonel Biesel and also talked with him in person and was told that no other "coats" had reported having any similar problem.

I was in anesthesia school in 1985 in Washington , D.C. and attended part of the reunion at that time, I missed the Friday night session, but attended the Saturday program. By the way, I did not complete anesthesia school but still work as a Nurse and am presently transitioning into the financial services business.

Charles Martin

After having served in Singapore for nine years as Youth and National Service Organization director of the Far Eastern Division, I had the privilege of working as an associate in the same departments of the General Conference. Beginning in late 1966, I learned much I had not known previously about Project Whitecoat.

Selection of Whitecoat Volunteers

Having been out of the country for a rather long period, and even before that while working entirely on the West Coast, my knowledge of Whitecoat was very limited. As I learned more about the program, I found myself agreeing with it, appreciating its purposes, and doing all I could to support it. I was impressed with the manner in which the program was being carried out. The better acquainted I became with its activities, the more I began to value the quality of men involved, not only the servicemen themselves, but also the officers.

For instance, I remember my first few trips to Fort Sam Houston, Texas to assist with the selection of volunteers. At that time, the project commander was COL Dan Crozier and his deputy LTC Ostereich. Watching these men present the concepts of Whitecoat to the draftees at Fort Sam, and seeing the serious attempt to make the program as clear as possible, was refreshing. I especially appreciated the careful effort to accept only those men who volunteered for the project. There was no arm-twisting or pressure.

As church representative for these selections, either Clark Smith or I assured the men involved that the church approved of the program, but that it was completely their decision if they wished to sign up. We emphasized the fact that we were there to guide and assist. Not only did the men have to volunteer to enter the program, but they also had to volunteer for every protocol in which they would be involved.

The New Servicemen's Center

As the program continued, more and more Whitecoat volunteers moved into the Washington, D.C. area, some stationed at Fort Detrick, near Frederick, and some assigned to the Walter Reed unit at Forest Glen. It soon became apparent that some type of servicemen's center would have to be established to care for their needs. So the Youth/National Service Organization Department leaders met with General Conference officer's to lay plans. Soon a young Adventist architect in Takoma Park, Buddy Hart, was assigned to the project. The building plans were finalized, construction got under way, and in good time a modern, attractive center was completed. It was Tom Green, the new center director, and his wife Priscilla, who added the home-like touch and made it a favorite spot for the men of Operation Whitecoat.

The dedication of the new Takoma Park Servicemen's Center was a special occasion. The featured speaker was Chaplain Major General Sampson, Chief Chaplain, U.S. Army, and special guests included not only General Conference leaders and other church workers, but also a large group of Whitecoat volunteers.

Speaking of care given the men of Whitecoat, a special tribute needs to be given to the Frederick SDA church. For years this congregation provided interest, care, and support for allWhitecoat members. Located near Fort Detrick in Maryland, this church gave special help to those men and families nearby during the entire time the program was in operation. After the Whitecoat program was terminated when the draft ended, the Frederick church has continued to host Whitecoat reunions periodically, and these have meant much to all members and their families.

There Were Some Rough Times

Throughout it's entire existence, Project Whitecoat had the loyal support of church leadership. Certainly there were questions asked; some groups raised objections to the church's involvement in such a program. The public media even got involved, especially during the days of the antiwar, anti-government activities.

I remember the visit to the General Conference by Seymour Hersch, a reporter from the Washington Post (later he was employed by the New York *Times* and subsequently became a Pulitzer Prize winner). This was during the days of America's involvement in Vietnam and the time of youth demonstrations. Hersch felt he had a real story; a church directly involved with the military in a questionable relationship. He telephoned our office, requesting an interview. This was arranged, and on the designated day Clark Smith and I, along with other available members of the National Service Organization Committee (a number of them General Conference officers), assembled in the committee room on the first floor of the old central General Conference building.

Hersch brought in his questions. From the beginning it was apparent that many of them were slanted, others loaded. Soon all realized that he had come with a specific agenda and wanted the interview to go in just one direction. Our church officials were frank and open, presenting information asked for, with data to back up the answers. Considerable research had been done and the information was freely given to Mr. Hersch. Whitecoat's objectives and goals were presented, and a clear description was given of the church's activities in the program. At the close of the interview it appeared that Hersch had received the facts desired and we felt some good might come of all this.

Consequently, a couple of days later all of us were shocked when we saw his article as it appeared in a prominent place in the Post. Rather than presenting a fair and accurate picture of Project Whitecoat, the description was mainly negative. Facts were distorted and twisted, portions of the material were actually falsified, and key positive parts of the program were not even mentioned. Needless to say, it took some time to clear the air and have the actual story of Whitecoat's accomplishments understood.

This experience rather vividly reflected the atmosphere which seemed to prevail across the country during those anti-war years. But through it all Project Whitecoat moved ahead, making a real contribution.

In Retrospect

Looking back on the Whitecoat chapter of the Adventist Church, one will find many pleasant and positive results. Not only were many of our church members able to fulfill their military obligation, as loyal citizens, but they were also able to make a meaningful contribution to medical science. This program provided an unusual opportunity for Seventh-day Adventists, with our strong belief in the health message, to demonstrate in a meaningful way our desire to serve our fellow men.

David B. Crooker

I was stationed at Fort Detrick as a lab assistant to Dr. Michael Kehoe, along with Ronald Lambeth, Rudy Richli and Robert Arthur (also Whitecoat volunteers), and Mary Thompson and William Thompson, civilian employees. A paper on our work was published in *The Journal of Infectious Diseases* in October, 1969.

I was involved in one "project." This was a two-week test of Eastern Equine Encephalitis (EEE) vaccine conducted in July, 1967. Prior to the project, each volunteer was interviewed individually by COL Crozier and other staff members, provided a complete explanation of the project, and given an opportunity to ask questions. There was no coercion whatsoever. Participation in each individual project was completely voluntary. It was entirely possible to enter Operation Whitecoat and never be part of an experiment.

I look back on my participation in Operation Whitecoat with a lot of pride in the contributions this program has made to the basic understanding of infectious diseases and the safeguards developed for our armed forces, which have been applied as recently as Desert Storm. There will always be those who are opposed to projects such as this, and the high tech and somewhat secretive nature of the work only adds to speculation and rumors.

I toured the USAMRIID facilities in September, 1989 as part of the second Whitecoat reunion. I was very impressed by the openness of the Army personnel in discussing the nature of the work, both historic and current, including offensive germ warfare development in the past. If the book is candid in discussing these issues also, it will go a long way toward putting some of the negative connotations of Operation Whitecoat in proper perspective.

Roy C. Culler

When I joined the Medical Research Institute in 1966 as the Chief Engineer, responsible for the research building's utilities servers, I had no idea how my life would change.

Gerald Rockwell, my first Whitecoat, was assigned to my office in 1969. Following is a list some of the Whitecoats assigned to the engineering section in the ensuing years: Gerald Rockwell, Roland Mays, Everett Blair, Harold Burgeson, Jeffrey Rice, Gary Swanson Ronald Koistad, Robert Wolfe, Buford Fry, Philip Castleburg, Eldon Jensen, Randall Tarzswell, Douglas Martin, Douglas Schroeder, Kenneth Sanders, James Mann, Dale Hainey, Claire Erickson, Michael Conger, Dwight Newbold, Wayne Lee, Robert Kaiser, Edward Vance, Ronald Wood, David Van Gundy, James Aldred, Randall Rima, Alvarado Gonzales, Eugene Burtneff, Larry Bowies, Kenneth Cobb, Scott Shipman, Ronald Winslow, Robert Claybum, Donald Park, Daniel Lawing, Michael Keyser, Glen Garver, Jim Harboffle, Joe Milfeit, Wayne Berg, David Kratzer, John Steinbeck, Larry Chadwell, Joe Sindoni, Shannon Giatt, Leroy Byers, Dale Cruffenden, Heine Wiegand.

All of the men came from good families, had finished college, or had one to two years to complete. I found them to be responsible men who took their jobs seriously and kept the building in good, clean condition. Most men were compatible with each other, and being in the Army kept personal conflicts to a minimum. They were a joy to work with and a rare group of men.

During the years after the draft was abolished, the new breed of volunteers were court cases, uneducated, undependable misfits who needed constant supervision. It was a demanding task to get them to complete assignments and do them correctly, a task I was not accustomed to with the Whitecoats.

Tarzswell reenlisted several times, serving eight years with the office. I have been able to keep in touch with Tarzswell, and many times I have wished I could locate more, especially Rockwell. Of the fifteen years I worked at the Institute prior to my retirement, the first eight years, I am proud to say, were the most memorable of my career.

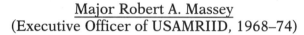

Major Robert A. Massey
(Executive Officer of USAMRIID, 1968–74)

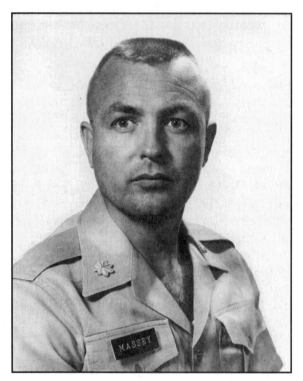

I recall the enthusiasm of COL Crozier with the construction of the new USAMRIID and the significantly improved design of the Volunteer Ward, not only for the enhancement of studies, but for the basic personal comforts for the Whitecoats. His enthusiasm was contagious and his dream for a comfortable and pleasing restricted hospitalization area were realized. He wanted each volunteer to have a clean, sterile, comfortable room with an outside view, and he achieved that. He also insisted on comfortable surroundings for visiting purposes, and installed a phone for private conversations between husband and wife or guests of Whitecoats. He also insisted on a pleasant recreation area even though they might not use it during their "sick time" while in the hospital. His overall concern was for their physical and emotional health while participating in a study. "Informed consent" requirements of all project protocols was another insistence of the Colonel's. I would expect that the Whitecoats might have many stories regarding the explanations by Doctors Peter Bartelloni and Frank Calia; such an important but difficult issue to cover with potential study volunteers. However, it was done to the letter of the law.

It goes without saying that the Company Commander's job was much less demanding (comparatively speaking) from the standpoint of disciplinary control and much more rewarding because of the Company's achievements. In my opinion, the Whitecoat population was personally disciplined and behaviorally mature and responsible. Article 15 administration was rare, and I do not recall there ever being a court martial (UCMJ administration) during the period in discussion.

In our recruitment trips to Fort Sam (normally made with COL Crozier and Elder Smith, and on occasion, Elder Martin), we always conducted an occupational skills manpower need of our operating divisions and endeavored to identify the number and types of studies to be conducted. Selections were generally difficult, for there was so much talent to choose from. Needless to say, if any of the potential Whitecoats had avocational talents in any physical sport, it did not work against them. It was viewed as another outlet for effectively dealing with the special assignments for which they were volunteering.

Coincidentally, and on the lighter side, I don't recall our not winning the Commander's sports trophy during my tenure. We tended to acquire the most points each year in the various competitions between the companies to earn the honor of the Commander's trophy — primarily attributable to our Whitecoats. Some names come to mind, such as Pangman (softball pitcher), Hoffman (touch football), Willy (touch football). This was the time of Vietnam and Willy (I believe it was Willy), who was also the CLS's driver, volunteered to go to RVN [Republic of Vietnam] for duty as a medic; I understand he served admirably.

I remember that motorcycles were a hot item. It was very difficult to discourage men at that age to avoid them, or to at least use them with extreme caution. Unfortunately, a tragic personal experience was the real teacher. I believe it was Hoffman, Willy, and a couple of others who went out to lunch on their cycles. I really believe that it wasn't horse play, but Hoffman wound up skidding on the sand on a back road into a barbed wire fence, pealing the skin off his neck from carotid artery to carotid artery. This slowed down the motorcycle fad for a while.

Food was always a critical issue. There was constant liaison with the Consolidated Mess staff to ensure that there was adequate vegetable selection and portions. In spite of our vigilance, my guess is that this may have been one of the most difficult situations for the men to deal with.

I recall the unfortunate incident of the shootout in the mess hall; no Whitecoat involvement. One of the soldiers really went on a rampage over a marital issue (wife was in Frederick, but he was assigned elsewhere). He wound up killing a few innocent soldiers. I would assume it was a memorable event for those assigned at that time.

My opinion is that we had the best in First Sergeants and Sergeant Majors at the time. Both Dave Shoop and George Leggins were top-notch and truly concerned about the health, morale and welfare of the Whitecoats, and most proud of their accomplishments. A limited number of Whitecoats got tertiary authorship for some professional articles written for studies that they worked on very closely with their Research Scientists.

A tremendously musically-inclined Whitecoat, I believe Buzz Sterreft (sp. ?), offered another outlet via the musical mode. It was not only healthy routine activity, but also healthy while under the stress of projects. We were able to provide limited instruments for use during the studies, and kept them tuned by allowing their use during off-study time. Along this same line, I recall a member by the name of "Moon" who was a skilled pianist. He offered another much appreciated dimension to the chapel in his services as a chaplain's assistant.

Maybe some of the Whitecoats would share some personal experiences regarding our liaisons with Hood College. I recall that we appeared to be high on the Hood College students' interest and "invite list" for their activities.

The Washington, D.C. area was a high cost of living area. It goes without saying that the retreat area offered by the church, with Elder Green in charge, offered a comforting home away from home for the Whitecoats stationed in the D.C. area. I remember the enthusiasm of Pastor White, who was so conscientiously working to duplicate the D.C. facility concept in the Frederick area. The unexpected change in the draft during this time may have precluded its paralleling the services for Frederick Whitecoats to those offered in D.C. However, it appears that his early efforts were most effectively redirected for an invaluable use.

When we moved to the new research building, we had one of the most farsighted facilities at the time. It also meant that the maintenance function was critical and sophisticated to accommodate the 26 special containment laboratories. Those Whitecoats who were blessed with maintenance interests and skills were tremendously rewarded by their work experiences with Roy Culler. We had one of the first-generation computer programs for monitoring and identifying geographical problem areas in the building. Varga's name seems to stand out in my mind for some reason.

Finally, I remember Mr. Zimmerman, Deputy Comptroller, WRAMC, always being so thankful to have such talented and financially capable volunteers to work on special comptroller projects. Generally, this was a universal feeling of supervisor's of the Whitecoats assigned to the Washington area.

Sgt. Francis W. Sexton

(Francis Sexton was a noncommissioned officer in the Physical Science Division, responsible for research equipment, operation of the laboratory, and the training of research assistants.)

When I first reported to the U.S. Army Medical Unit at Fort Detrick, I was totally unprepared for the lack of military appearance of the troops. They were nothing like the Army personnel I was accustomed to. There was an absence of military bearing or discipline. My unit in Japan had not been noted for its military appearance, but it looked like a unit of West Point cadets by comparison. It took about six months for me to adapt to this lack of military conduct, and it wasn't easy. The 1st Sergeant explained to me that these were mostly volunteers for medical research, and they were not to be expected to perform like regular soldiers. Neither were they to be harassed or coerced in any way. They were expected to be trained into whatever duties we could find for them, but those duties were secondary to their primary function as medical volunteers.

The men were from a wide range of educational backgrounds. Some held degrees, while others may not have completed high school. For the most part, I found that they were dedicated to their beliefs and were prepared to perform the very special duty for which they had volunteered. We were able to train them to perform many different jobs, such as medical laboratory technicians, medical research technicians, hospital corpsmen, animal handlers and technicians, and a score of other positions. These positions occupied their time when they weren't on a project. Since there were so few regular Army enlisted cadre in the unit, these men did most of the day-to-day duties of a medical research unit. There were times when a man had to be transferred from one duty to another for various reasons, but for the most part they performed well.

The men were used to test vaccines for the military. These vaccines had passed all the necessary animal tests and had to pass the final test, the human one. Very careful watch was kept on those volunteers who were in a vaccine test. Blood tests were done, temperatures taken, physical exams repeated, and other procedures done throughout the entire time of the test. At no time was there a period when they were not checked and rechecked. After a test was over, special leave was granted, but blood tests had to be drawn during leave and the volunteers were given instructions to return to the unit if anything unusual occurred with their health. Also, special care was taken to insure that not too much blood was drawn during a project. Total blood requirement for the project was calculated, and if it appeared that an excess was wanted, then the project was modified to reduce the amount.

Two projects stick in my mind, neither related to vaccines. One project was on human diurnal variation and the other was on operation of complicated equipment while ill. The diurnal variation project consisted of establishing a baseline of physical levels, with testing around the clock and for regular daytime activity for about two weeks. Then we reversed the schedule so that all regular activity took place during the normal resting hours; that is, we reversed the entire living schedule from day to night and night to day. This was maintained for about two weeks. The body function tests showed that humans possessed diurnal variation, while rats do not. This had implications as to when medications and treatments should be given.

Another fact that was discovered, quite by accident during routine testing of Yellow Fever vaccine, was that the coagulation time of blood was longer for a day or two after a Yellow Fever inoculation was given. Personnel who were given Yellow Fever shots just prior to engaging in combat, if wounded might require more whole blood or blood-volume extenders due to an extended bleeding time.

There was also a project to determine how sick an equipment operator could become before he could no longer control his equipment. Mock control boards were brought in and volunteers were trained in their operation. Operational commands were received through earphones, equipment was operated, and compliance results were sent through microphones. After the volunteers were trained, they were given a very mild disease which simulated a cold or the flu. They then worked the controls in four-hour shifts. As their temperatures rose and the disease progressed, it became harder and harder for them to operate the proper control when the order was received. Finally they reached a stage where they could no longer operate the control boards. As soon as this stage was determined, all the volunteers were treated with the proper medication and returned to normal health in a day or two. There were no lasting effects, and NASA now knew when they would have to terminate a mission should the astronauts become ill during a flight.

The information gained from the volunteers was invaluable. However, since it was all classified, they never received recognition for their labors. No awards or medals were given, not even letters of appreciation or citations. In fact, it was even difficult to get promotions for them.

I went to Walter Reed Hospital once a month as a member of the lower promotion board. The Post sergeant major would complain to me that the "Detrick boys always look bad;" that they had no knowledge of Army weapons or traditions. It didn't surprise me, in that they had to drive a dusty bus down to Walter Reed, wait in the troop day room until the promotion board began, had no chance to press their uniforms or tidy up, and had little or no training in Army weapons or tradition. Going up against troops stationed at the Post did make them look bad. The Military Police always appeared in their black leather belts, white hats and polished holster's, and the Post medics were able to iron their uniforms just prior to the board.

After a discussion with the sergeant major and the medical detachment's 1st Sergeant, we got permission to have some cleaning and pressing equipment available in the day room. Also, a long talk about what the duties of a Whitecoat were, and what their training was, led to more understanding as to what these men did. It seemed to bring a bit more respect for personnel who were considered less than regular troops because they were conscientious objectors and were not regular Army draftees. Personally, I felt that the work they were doing was just as important, maybe even more important, than that being done by the average GI, and that some form of recognition should have been given. However, this was never done to my knowledge, except for a single soldier's work in development of electrophoresis stains, which was mentioned in a published paper.

I was also a member of the Post Soldier of the Month Board, and heard comments being made about the Commanding Officers in the Medical Unit, and how they couldn't answer weapons questions correctly. Again, a little talk about what they were and what they did helped. Many of the other unit NCOs [Non-Commissioned Officers] didn't know what was being done at the Army Medical Unit. They thought that these were regular Army medical personnel engaged in some secret work, similar to the Chemical Corps laboratory technicians who also worked on the Post.

I was greatly impressed by the elders of their church, who frequently came to the Post. They were a great help to the men and also to the NCOS. If we had a problem with one of the volunteers, the elders would help us work it out. Sometimes it was a simple military problem, but often it would involve parents, girlfriends or religious questions about diets, activities or worship time. The elders never failed to jump in and give of their time and knowledge. There were very few problems that were not solved in some way. As I recall, there were very few serious disciplinary actions taken against the volunteers.

My personal impression was that these were very involved young men, whose convictions did not allow them to bear arms, but who wanted to do something for their country. Their contributions were immense, but can't really be measured. I feel sure that there might have been some men not as dedicated as others, but that would be expected in any group of military personnel. Overall, I think that the Whitecoats performed a very important service for the United States and were never officially recognized for that service. However, unfortunately this is only my opinion, and not that of the military or of the government.

Doris Blood

The first recollection I have of the Whitecoats in Frederick was about 1955. Elder David and Doris Miller were here as our Pastor, with their children Alice and Bobby. Many were the Saturday nights that we would spend at their home singing and playing games. Their home was always open to everyone. Many of the GIs would also come over for a fun-filled evening. It was always a standing joke that Elder Miller lived between two "beer joints" and Jefferson Street.

There are only three names I can think of from 1955: Don Johnson, Art Blake, and Wendall Parish. Art played the saw. Wendall Parish was a good looking guy; my Daddy wouldn't let me near him. All the girls gave him a second look! Don't know what happened to him. Don Johnson is now a surgeon in California. Art Blake returned to Michigan. Also, there was a nice married couple, Bob and Arlene Lee. I believe they were from California. Bob played the steel guitar and Arlene played the piano. She also had a small keyboard organ that she attached to the piano. It added so much to our church services. Bob sold his steel guitar when he left. I wanted it, but was told I couldn't have anything else until I did more practicing on the piano. I was angry, but it did me no good. So Jimmy Bryant ended up with the guitar.

Quite a few of the fellows were coming to church. The church had been having dinners each week for them for some time. Many

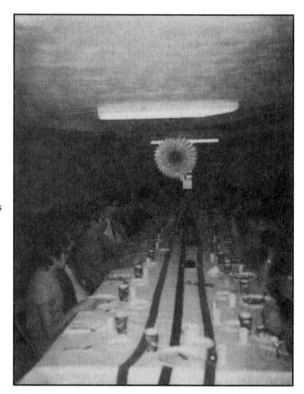

A Whitecoat Christmas Party in 1971.

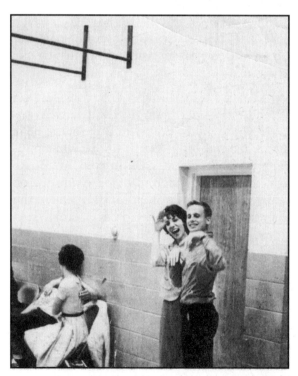

Skating (and the girls) were always popular with off-duty Whitecoats.

families joined in with the dinners. The guys would come to church knowing there would be a good dinner waiting. Before we started having the dinners, when they came to church, they would always miss their dinner at the barracks. Many of them participated in our Young Peoples Meetings on Friday nights as well as church services. Many sang and played musical instruments. We always had lots of special music; lots of Saturday night activities at the church. One Saturday evening, a girl friend from Walkersville High and I wanted to shop. The only big place then was the Seventh Street Shopping Center. Mom and Daddy decided they would visit the Elliotts from church while we shopped. Well, we ran into three of the guys and they had no car. They wanted to go to a snack bar, so off we went! I had Daddy's 1956 Mercury. Time slipped away and it was 10:30 p.m. when we returned to the Elliotts to pick up Mom and Daddy. Sure was glad to have Ruth with me; otherwise they may not have believed me.

From around 1955 until Daddy quit farming in 1965 or 1966, whenever we had a lot of hay to bring in, the guys would come out and help. We always gave them a good meal. I loved to cook even back then, so I had someone to practice on. There was a time they were puffing hay up in the barn and joking about how they felt the floor "give." The next morning it was no joke; the ceiling and all the hay were down in the cowbarn. There were no cows in the barn at the time, or it could have been much worse.

Our church membership was quite small at this time, with not many teenagers. A lot of the guys would go to Columbia Union College on Sabbaths. However, a number still stayed here in Frederick. Some of us ended up marrying GIs. I married Colis Blood on March 22, 1959. We had four servicemen in our wedding: Donald Begley as best man, Henry Surdal, Raymon Altizer, and Parker. Parker was a Catholic friend of Colis's; the rest were Adventists. They were just as bad for tin-canning cars then as they are now, so Colis hid the car. But while we were trying to get away from everyone I forgot my suitcase and had to come back. We lived in Betsy Ross Trailer Park until November 1961, at which time we moved to the farm. The guys came to Sabbath dinner there at the farm until Mom and Daddy moved in 1968 to Broadview Acres. While in the trailer park we would have guys come out on many Sabbaths.

Madode DeLong also married a serviceman, Kenneth Gaede, in June 1959 and moved to California, where she still resides. Jim Boodman spent many a Sabbath with us when Annette had to work at the hospital. A friend from Mt. Aetna Academy, Hollis (Pete) Viehmann (we graduated together), came into the service at this time and often spent Sabbath with us. He still visits and stays here on his trips back home. There was a guy whose last name was Davis who used to come to the trailer and bake us the best bread. He tried to teach me. I never did learn, but sure did enjoy his. He'd keep one loaf and we'd keep one loaf.

We continued to have the servicemen for dinner after we moved here in 1968. I had as many as 48 here in our home. I always have enjoyed cooking for anyone who wanted to come. I could try all kinds of new recipes on them and they seemed to enjoy.

We made many friends during Colis's service time (6 years). He spent 5 years at Detrick. There are quite a few we still hear from at Christmas and some who still visit from time to time. They know they are welcome here; we always find a spare bed or corner and there's always a spare key. One couple from Ohio goes on vacation with me every couple of years. Some of the best and longest lasting friendships I have, have come from our service friends. I have lots of places to vacation.

As a side note: On Sept. 14, 1962, Colis was to sing for young peoples' meeting that Friday. However, Pamie decided it was time for her to make her appearance. So we stopped at the church on the way to the hospital at 7:30 to tell them he couldn't sing. He went back at 9:00 to tell them he had a little 5 lb. daughter. The Warrens (a GI family) were expecting their first child. We had planned to be roommates. However, she was 3 weeks late. So much for careful planning.

Goldie and Byron Crum

We remember the years our servicemen were at Fort Detrick. They came to our home many times on Sabbath for dinner. I think at one time we had as many as 28 boys. They seemed to be very happy to get out to our farm in the country. We also enjoyed having them.

There were so many that I cannot remember all of their names, but I do remember a few special ones who used to come out in the summertime and help us get the hay into the barn. I remember Henry Surdal, who was extremely well built and very strong. He was raised on a farm, I believe in Montana. He was a very good worker. I remember other good farm workers: Carlin Cain, Don Begley, and John Eckland. There were others, but I can't remember all of their names.

I remember talking to one of them who came from the West. I remarked about our beautiful Blue Ridge Mountains being so pretty and high. He answered that our mountains were like mole hills to their's and then he laughed.

It surely would be nice to see them all again. We wish them all good health and good luck. God bless them all and their families. We loved them all.

Jane Damazo

The Frederick church initiated a program to make the young men coming into the area feel welcome, and with that a Sabbath meal was provided for all those who would care to come. These meals would be provided by the church members in their homes so we could get to know them on a personal basis.

Frederick County area is largely of German ancestry and it is impressed early on the minds that when you entertain folks, the appropriate amount of food must be served. It is a "sin" to do otherwise, and thus I identify with the biblical Martha. This story is about the one Sabbath dinner that will remain with me until the day I turn 100 plus 3 more days. It was our turn to entertain the servicemen and we had gotten a head count of 15 for dinner. I had stayed home that particular Sabbath with a small baby to make the last minute preparations. Everything was on schedule when the servicemen began to arrive, and as I was greeting them at the front door I turned to see my husband, Herb, coming from the back door followed by a large group of girls. He rushed in to tell me that he had invited 17 nursing students from the Washington Sanitarium and Hospital for dinner, and that they had made a special trip that morning to the Frederick church to look over the Adventist male prospects. He said they would not get a good opportunity to do this unless he invited them to dinner to get acquainted with the servicemen. He reassured me that food was not on their minds and that they would not realize that we did not have enough prepared. By now he was holding me up and telling me to smile. Though filled with panic (there is not enough Italian meat balls with sauce, rice or salad, etc.), I am smiling. It was quickly determined the house was not large enough to accommodate everybody, for by then we had a head count of 37 people for dinner. Well, you make the best of situations. We had a large freezer which was filled, and we went to work.

Folding chairs were brought over from the church and, we put the servicemen and nurses to work setting up the chairs outdoors, for it was a nice, sunny, spring day. I shall never forget what I saw. There they were setting up the chairs in neat rows, with the nurses lining their chairs up on one side of the sidewalk and the servicemen lining their chairs up on the opposite side of the sidewalk, directly facing each other. Both sides spent the next two hours looking each other over and generally having a good time getting acquainted. My husband, Herb Damazo, was right; food was not on their minds. Believe it or not, but there was at least one marriage from that day's encounter.

Ralph and Alberta Reed

Dear Chaplain Mole:

Doctor Frank Damazo has asked our family to write some recollections about our involvement in providing hospitality to the Whitecoats at Fort Detrick. But before I do, my husband thought you might enjoy some comments about his service time in the U.S. Navy. He was drafted in 1956 by the Army. When he was inducted, he was informed that he was being transferred to the Navy and would be sent to Bainbridge, Maryland. He had never been on the East Coast and wasn't really too sure where Maryland was.

Having entered the service as a conscientious objector, he had no idea what he would be facing when he reached Bainbridge. When he was being processed in at Bainbridge, he was called out of the line and told to follow one of the men. No explanations—just to follow that man! They went out of the building and got into a jeep and Ralph says he had no idea what was happening to him. The man drew up in front of a building and told him to go down the stairs and left him there to follow his instruction. When Ralph got inside the building, there was a man named Chaplain Robert Mole who met him and told him that a special company was being formed for the COs [consciences objectors] that would be trained as medics for the Navy, that he was an SDA chaplain, and that he had already arranged for this group to have Sabbath privileges.

Because Ralph had had Medical Cadet Corps training at Camp Carlyle B. Haynes in Colorado, he was made the recruit Chief Petty Officer and got to know you pretty well during his boot camp days and during the time his group stayed on at Bainbridge for Corps School. He still claims that he was never so glad to see anyone as he was to see you that day he arrived at Bainbridge. We look forward to seeing you at the next Whitecoat reunion in 1993 in Frederick.

When Ralph accepted the position of principal at the Frederick Church School in 1966, we really looked forward to moving to Frederick. We arrived wanting to be involved in the church's interface with the Whitecoats from Fort Detrick. We remembered all too well what it was like to be a long way from home when Ralph was in the Navy, and we also remembered a bad experience we had as visitors at an Adventist church. Ralph was stationed 70 miles from the nearest Adventist church and we didn't have a car. When we did purchase a car, we were so eager to go to church that we arranged for a long weekend and booked ourselves into a hotel.

When we arrived at the church, we felt ill at ease. We were told the church was between ministers, and they didn't seem too well organized. The worst part was that no one was friendly and we were starved for Adventist friendship. No one asked us our names, where we were from, or made any attempt to make us feel welcome. I will say that we had gone to church in civilian clothes, so there wasn't a visible clue we were service personnel. We wished later that we had just slept in at the hotel. We sure would have felt better in the long run. Needless to say, we never went back. We promised ourselves way back then that if we ever had service people visit a church where we were members, we'd go out of our way to make sure they felt welcome; never dreaming we'd end up in Frederick years later.

Our brother-in-law had been a Whitecoat at Fort Detrick before we moved to Frederick. When we told him we planned to get actively involved in inviting servicemen to our home, he encouraged us to include the married folks as well. It had been his observation that the GIs were struggling to make ends meet and that by the time the end of the month drew near, some of them were really hurting. So when it was our turn to have the GIs come to our home on Sabbath, we always prepared extra food so we could include several of the married couples as well.

Doctor Frank asked us to share some of the impact that our contact with the Whitecoat operation made on our lives. Every year at Christmas, we continue to hear from quite a few of the couples we grew to know and love while they were stationed at Fort Detrick. Just last week, we received an invitation to the wedding of one of the babies that was born while his Dad was on project for 30 days. Each year, we look forward to the letters and pictures from many of the couples, letting us know what has happened in their lives during that year, and we also keep them updated on what has happened in our lives.

When we arrived in Frederick, we had an eight year old daughter, whose name is Robin. Some of the couples "child sat" with her when Ralph and I needed to be at an appointment where children were not included. Before the Whitecoat operation came to an end, she was babysitting with some of their children. They played card games with her, Monopoly, checkers, etc. The fellow who taught her how to play Chinese Checkers is now a doctor serving in the mission field.

Recently, one of our Frederick church members who works at the General Conference was in the part of the world where their family is serving and the missionary wife was surprised to learn he lived in Frederick. She told him how she taught music at the church school and how our church had a baby shower for her, and when her husband was on duty or on project she would bring the baby and settle her in with our family while she played for the service. (Of course, this delighted Robin to help care for the baby.) The missionary wife told him about the Reed family and was surprised to learn we still live in Frederick. We had lost touch with them over the years, and were very pleased when our friend brought their greetings back to us.

We really got to know the couples who were willing to take an active part in our church. Some of them were quite musically talented and often I would accompany them. They would come out to our home on Friday night to practice and afterward would stay and visit with us. Several of the couples are still in our church. They either married local girls and decided to stay on after they finished their tour of duty, or in the case of one couple, they came back to Frederick to live. A sad note happened a few weeks ago when one of the GIs from Wyoming who married a local girl, lost his wife. This couple has been part of our church for 25 years, and while she was not an Adventist when he met her, she did join our church and has been a faithful member up until her death.

What makes it so nice is that from time to time, some of these GI couples come back to visit. During the two reunions, we have had the wonderful privilege of seeing many of them again. From time to time, they come back to the East Coast so that the children who were born here and those who were born later can see where Dad served in the military. During the years we got to meet some of the parents who came East to visit their children.

I head up the group who serve as host and hostesses (greeters) for our church. When they come, they usually write on their visitors' cards that they were a part of the Whitecoat operation. It tells me that they were proud to serve their country at Fort Detrick, but it also tells me that they have a very soft spot in their heart for the Frederick church. Many of our members opened their homes and made room in their hearts for these young people. For many, it was the first time to be so far from home and it didn't take too much entertaining on our parts to make them happy. They just wanted a place to come when they needed a substitute parent and to feel that someone did care what happened to them. Our church did not let them down. I think another wonderful part is to know where some of them are serving today and that they have stayed close to our Adventist church and our big Adventist family.

Royer Family

The following information is for the use of Chaplain Mole in the preparation of his book on the Whitecoats at Fort Detrick. This information is supplied by the Royer family because of our close association with the many of these young men.

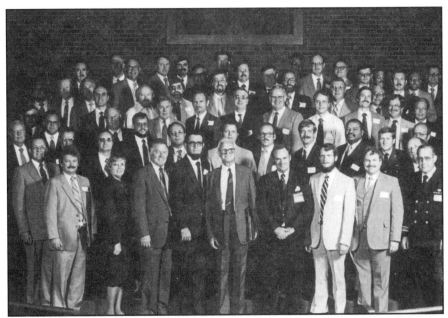

First Whitecoat reunion in September, 1985. Colonel Crozier is in the center of the front row.

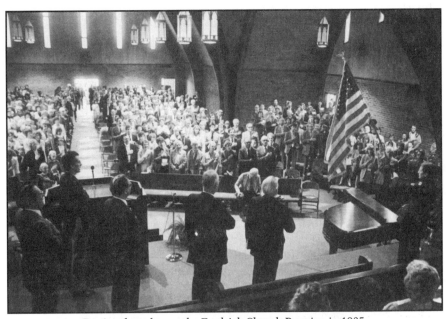

Posting the colors at the Fredrick Church Reunion in 1985.

My first recollection of any Adventist soldier at Fort Detrick was in 1953. In those days very few soldiers of the Adventist faith were stationed at Detrick and they were not called Whitecoats. Most of these men were married with families of their own and not necessarily living on the Post. The first one whose name I remember was Davis; he aspired to become a dentist. From that time on I didn't have much contact with Adventists on the Post until the beginning of the Vietnam conflict.

When the first Whitecoats started to come into Fort Detrick, the Army tired to utilize their services but at the same time realized that they had a problem with these young men in that their diet was different and their way of living was different. The Army tried hard to see that these young men were fed properly and had proper recreation, but until they became efficient at it the boys suffered a bit in that they had to go elsewhere for food to supplement their diet. The church recognized the need of supplying food and entertainment for these young men and they used the auditorium of our new school for the area to entertain and feed them. The families would go together to prepare the food. We played volleyball and track games, roller-skated, and did other things in the auditorium. They would usually feed pizzas supplied by the Reed family. Ralph used to bake them in special ovens that we had acquired for that purpose. The boys would scatter from there and go to other places.

As these things usually happen, certain groups would pick up with different families and visit them more than they would others. This is how we became involved with a certain group of these young men. The first group that I remember was the older men, in their twenties. The first ones of those was Duff Stoltz, Allen Roth, David Moody, John Ashford, and a few other's whose names I cannot recall. These young men would be out there almost every evening, Sabbath afternoons, and Sundays. We would feed them according to the season.

We owned a small farm in a very remote area of Frederick County and we produced our own vegetables and fruits. We canned and froze a lot, so we always had plenty of food on hand. They would come and enjoy the television programs, and would stay until the wee hours of the morning. When they would leave they would lock the house and go on home, as we family members had already gone to bed. Next day they would be back.

It was a delight to have these young men; they treated our children as if they were their own brothers and sisters and we treated them as family. That is what these young men enjoyed more than anything else because they were all so lonely. The environment that they had for recreation at Fort Detrick was such that they just couldn't adapt to it. The recreation rooms would be full of tobacco smoke and the fellows would be drinking and the language would be different than these young men used; so you can see why they were anxious to get away.

As each group would leave the service a new group would come and take their place. Of course the word got around where the best places to go were, and since we lived where we did and we were in very close proximity to Harpers Ferry and places like that in the mountain areas, we received, I dare say, the bulk of the men.

In the fall of the year we would always have fruit pies, pumpkin pies, cakes, Adventist food, of course, and root beer and fresh cider. The fellows enjoyed this, and they would quite often bring their friends and relatives out to visit when they were near Frederick. Often they would go to Washington, D.C., Walter Reed, Forest Glen and places like that, and they would take our children with them—as many as they could get in the car. They would tour Washington and then come back and stay at the house for a while.

One evening, one of the soldiers, an Armenian named Ed Khanoyan, brought out his entire family, who had come for a visit. It was winter and in the area we lived, a severe snow storm or blizzard might drift us in, sometimes for a week or two weeks at a time. The only way out was to walk up to the main road. We had become used to that and quite often we would just park our vehicle on the main road and walk up to the house because some of those drifts on the dirt roads could be fifteen feet high and quite often would drift shut. The only way to open them was to come in with bulldozers and just push it out. Well, it started to snow that afternoon and Ed wanted to stay overnight, to get snowed in. Of course he didn't know what being snowed in was, but he wanted to be snowed in. We finally persuaded him he'd better leave because if he got snowed in he wasn't going to get out for a while. They did leave, but on the way back to Washington it got so bad that something happened to their car; they had to call the chaplain from the Forest Glen area, who came out with several automobiles to rescue them. Things like that were happening throughout.

I remember one party we had; there were between thirty and forty GIs in our home at the same time—there wasn't room for them to be around the periphery of the living room. They played music, sang songs, told jokes and stories about their home, and played a few parlor games. They really enjoyed themselves. Another time a big group came out for a party in the evening. It happened to be a nice, balmy, late spring evening with a bright moon. There were over 300 acres of farmland to roam over. The ground in this area where we were is quite hilly, with many ravines grown up in brush and trees; it was heavily wooded as well as pastureland. They decided that they were going to play a version of hide and seek. They split up into teams and went out over this acreage and then they proceeded to try to find each other. They could run from hill to hill and from field to field, and all the time they are doing this they were making all sorts of weird, screechy noises and just having a ball hollering, yelling and carrying on.

My second oldest daughter and Mr. Moser's son, who owned one of the farms that they were running over, were teamed up with one of the groups. Unbeknownst to these fellows, Dave Fisher and Cormola had brought along an amplifier on which they had placed a predator call—of a mountain lion. Every now and then they would turn this on and up the amplification on it. It made an awful, weird noise which would resound up and down that valley that you wouldn't believe. This went on until close to one o'clock in the morning.

They all had to come back across a little stream to get to our house, crossing what was called a high water bridge. Rick and Lynn were together, and as they got out on the cement part of the bridge, Comola opened up his amplifier again and let out a couple of loud screeches. Of course Lynn tired to climb Rick and Rick tried to climb Lynn and they were all tangled up and wrestling with each other and trying to run and couldn't. Everybody got a big charge out of it.

The next morning as I was going up to Jefferson, my neighbor, John Whitlock, stopped me. He owned the farm that was up the stream from us, and joining Moser's. He said to me "Bill, did you hear that awful racket last night; that unearthly caterwauling. I was really frightened. I thought there was something in my cattle out in the fields and trying to kill them. I got my rifle and went out to look. I couldn't see or hear anything. I could hardly sleep all night long. I was just scared to death." I laughed and told him what it was. He said "Man, the next time they do that, please let me know so I can go to bed. I won't have to worry. That was an awful sound." I imagine it was; but they had fun that night.

Another time we had planned a party for New Years Eve, 1965. Everything was ready to go. That morning my wife and I left to go to Frederick. I had to go to Fort Detrick and she was working as a nurse at the time, I believe. We got as far as Log Cabin Hill on old Route 340. A drunk had passed out behind the wheel of his car and had fallen over on the seat; he wasn't even in sight behind the wheel. He crossed the center line of the highway and hit us head on. Totally demolished both cars. I had just bought a brand new Mercury station wagon; had 400 miles on it; it was a total loss. Both of us were in the hospital for over two weeks. My wife had her cheek cut off and hanging, and glass in her eyes because her head went through the windshield and came back through it again. I had a broken sternum and my ribs were broken.

The boys decided to visit us each night. The first night they came by, they came marching in. There must have been about fifteen of them in the group. The nurses hadn't coped with anything like this before and they just didn't know what to do. When they found out who these boys were going to visit they came into the room and said, "What are we going to do?" The gentlemen who was in the room with me said "Just let those boys all come in here and stand and sit because we just love company and we would love to have them." He said to just let them come in and sit, so they could go out in groups to visit my wife because the lady she was sharing a room with didn't want anyone in the room, including another patient. Later on they changed her to a different room so these fellows could visit.

They visited us faithfully for two weeks and even took care of our children while we were away. Our oldest daughter was working for the County Commissioners at that time and the boys looked after the children. So we didn't have the party that night, but we found we had a lot of friends in the Whitecoats.

Some of the families who worked with these young men were the Crums, Carbaughs, Jones, Damazos, Royers and Reeds. The Carbaughs had horses and let the fellows ride. They would have parties in the barn and sit on bales of hay and play all sorts of games, especially around Halloween. They loved that. We would furnish homemade root beer and other refreshments for them. Our family would take them on trips around the area, to the mountains and what have you. The Damazos furnished a lot of food. The Reeds worked in the school and furnished facilities there. All in all the boys had a pretty good time of it.

Now I am going to give you some of the recollections that my second oldest daughter remembers. You must remember that these young men volunteered to be guinea pigs. The Army used them to test their inoculations and vaccinations and things like that on them. Of course some of them got quite ill. They had no fatalities, but this is what they submitted themselves to in order to serve their time in the Army for the Vietnam conflict. Lynn says that she remembers, starting in 1959, having Duff Stoltz, Allen Roth, David Moody and John Ashford come out to the house to visit. They were in their twenties and she was thirteen, and she looked at them as her older brothers. Then she remembers going mushroom hunting with a young man from the Northwest who drove a real antique car. She doesn't remember his name, but he taught her how to fry cheese and mushrooms. It really was delicious. They had parties at the Marvels, Marquinas and the Royers, playing games such as Gossip, Meow, Squirrel in the Tree, and going for long walks at night across our land and the neighbors' with a large group of young people. She remembers having Gary Strang sing for her on Sabbath afternoon; especially her favorite, "There were Ninety and Nine."

She remembers being captured on film more times than she can remember because every one of these boys was a shutterbug. They never missed an opportunity to take pictures of people and places; they were always snapping pictures. She has a special remembrance of Johnny Cruz who was from Puerto Rico; he gave her a special Bible. And she remembers sitting by the Fort Detrick pool and comparing suntans with Shannon Goodwin, a very nice young man. He was black and she was white, but she was always darker. He brought his wife out to visit us just before they were to be married in New York. He invited us to come up to New York for the wedding, but we couldn't make it. Shannon is the one who was on a show in New York. He was in the audience when one of the members of the Catholic Church, one of the well known bishops, was there speaking about Biblical facts. I think he had taken a trip to the Holy Land or something, and he was talking about it. He made some statements from the Bible that weren't accurate, and Shannon asked him about it. He said to Shannon, "Well, young man, I'll have to check when I go back since I don't have my Bible with me." Shannon said, "That's all right, I have mine. It's in my pocket." I don't know what came of it, but in any event that's what happened.

She remembers some of the guys who would come out and get snowed in occasionally. Then there were the barn parties at the Carbaughs'. Frank Sittig, who was from Oregon, used to love the homemade root beer. He could drink a whole quart of it at a time. He really enjoyed it. They would make and deliver apple pies to Carl Coffey and Lonnie Fultz while they were on project. I think they broke a few rules because they were in restricted areas, wards, and they may have been visiting where they shouldn't have been, but they got away with it.

Some of these boys have been back to see us. Allen Roth came back to see us not too long ago. Lonnie Fultz has been back twice as well as several of the other fellows that we met. They remember playing Monopoly to all hours with Dave Fisher, Bob Bowen, Lloyd Gibson and Dick Comola—also playing Pit with these guys when Bob had a cast on his elbow. Lynn remembers being thrown in the creek by Dave Strong. It was an accident, of course. A good thing it was summer. She spent many Sabbath afternoons over a period of years walking around Harpers Ferry with various fellows after a big lunch at home. There was always a good-sized group on these excursions.

She remembers making and eating popcorn pretty near every Sunday night for years, and she said she learned from the guys that it was good with Smokene or cheese on it—but she doesn't eat popcorn anymore! She says she visited the guys while they were on project, praying and worrying for some who became quite ill—such as Lonnie Fultz and Bob Visser. Many of them did become quite ill. She was the recipient of many homemade gifts by these fellows on project. They used to make pictures and butterflies and things out of mosaics and gilt and stones and such as that, and they were really quite attractive. She received pet nicknames from some of the guys. Her favorite nickname was Angel. She spent many wonderful times with Terry Cadisle, Bill Fentress and Jerry Shoemake, driving in the "Blue Bomb" or just walking and talking.

They used to watch the sun come up and then go out to breakfast with Paul Betlunski, Louis Vasquez, Terry Calisle and their dates. Louis married the daughter of Mr. Moser. Lynn used to go motorcycle riding through the country with Ron Lambeth. The first time she rode on a motorcycle she was with Louie Kintz. They were leaving a nursing home after having a "singspiration" there. The ride was short since she was still dressed in Sabbath clothes. While going on a drive in her new car, chauffeuring some of the guys, Dennis Smith was sitting in the front passenger seat. They were driving up a hill and going around a steep curve at the same time; there was a straight drop-off down to the creek on the passenger side, and she scared Dennis to death when she said she couldn't see the road anymore.

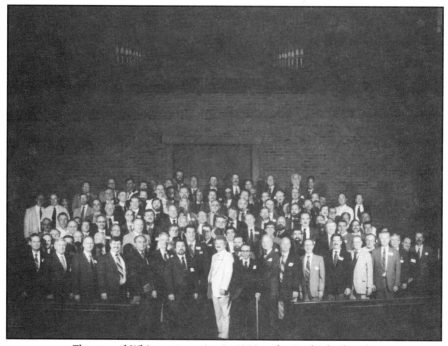

The second Whitecoat reunion in 1989 at the Fredrick Church.

They had many challenging games of volleyball in the school gym. Some guys played for blood, but most played for fun, clowning and chowing down later on red velvet cake or cookies that one of the girls had made, just for volleyball night. Roller skating in the gym on Saturday nights with Jerry Penner, Dave Strong, Danny Campbell and last, but definitely not least, her then future husband, Bob Cooke, is another memory. (Bob is an auditor now with the General Conference.) She also remembers piling into Ralph Wood's Volkswagen with about six or seven others and heading out for pizza. Talking on the phone for hours with one guy after another—they would line up to talk. That was when these guys would be on the ward. They were in for a project and they couldn't go anywhere, so they would line up to talk to somebody at home.

Then one time our dog had been hurt. We think it had been shot. There was a hole through its body below the backbone; but it didn't hit the spine. He was in pretty bad shape. Cad Coffey took him out to the Fort Detrick veterinarian. The wound healed up real nice and the dog got well.

These recollections are reflected by the whole family. We hope that you can use this information. Feel free to use it as you see fit. The names that we have mentioned here are not all of these young men that we knew by any means, but they are those that were the closest to us and were around most of the time. I wish you well on your book and I would like very much to be able to read it when you are finished with it.

OPERATION WHITECOAT

Reflections of Chaplain Tom Green

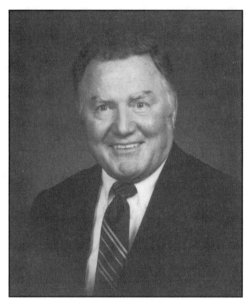

Chaplain Tom Green
Photo by Olan Mills

I have been asked to set down memories of my association with the Army medical research program called "Operation White-coat." It has now been over 30 years (November 1961) since I received a call from the Columbia Union Conference to serve as civilian chaplain in the Washington, D.C. area.

I was pastor of the Newark, New Jersey church at the time, having begun my ministry in the New Jersey Conference in 1951. I had served in several pastoral assignments, but was very active in the conference summer youth camps. It was for that reason Elder Ed Peterson, Columbia Union Conference Youth Director and National Service Organization Secretary, observed my work with young people and saw fit to recommend me for the role of civilian chaplain.

The reason the Church chose to station a civilian chaplain there was not only the large number of military bases nearby, but because of the Army research unit at Fort Detrick in Frederick, Maryland which was using large numbers of Seventh-day Adventist soldiers to staff unit jobs and to participate in research projects.

The program began recruiting Adventist 1–A–Os as early as 1955 from the Army Medical training center at Fort Sam Houston in San Antonio, Texas. It was not until 1959, however, that Edwin Reading was asked to serve as civilian chaplain for the Washington area. It was considered a part-time assignment for him while he was taking graduate work at Potomac University (the predecessor to Andrews University).

In 1961, when Ed Reading resigned from the task, church officials determined the need to replace him with a full-time civilian chaplain and the call was extended to me.

It has been over 30 years, but I still recall the elation in being afforded the opportunity to minister to Seventh-day Adventist young people in military service.

I had been an 18-year-old draftee in the latter days of World War II and I recalled how meaningful it had been to me when warm hearted church members reached out with kindness and hospitality at a time in my life when I could easily have drifted.

I thought perhaps my wife and I could serve as representatives of the church who would provide caring and non-judgmental acceptance to a lot of youth in uniform who were at a sensitive time of transition in their lives when many important decisions were being formed regarding faith, career, and marriage.

Time served to confirm that early assessment. I still regard the nearly 12 years we spent in that assignment as a unique opportunity to touch young lives in a significant way for good.

Moving to Takoma Park was a return home for me. My family originally moved there in 1939. We found the Seventh-day Adventist Church as a result of friendly neighbors inviting us to some meetings held by Francis D. Nichol and Terrance K. Martin from the Review and Herald.

I had gone to academy and college in Takoma Park and met my wife there. I had worked several years as a student in the Review and Herald bindery and had many friends in the area.

We bought a home just across the street from Dr. Ted Flaiz who was one of the key persons involved in the original negotiations concerning Operation Whitecoat. Our initial challenge was to find ways to reach the Adventist military personnel charged to our care. I ran across some notes I made early on of methods to try as we plunged into our task:

1. Obtain lists of names and information about military personnel in area. (The Whitecoat unit was very helpful in supplying rosters and lists of incoming troops.)

2. Visit and talk with service personnel and families.

3. Devise ways to help incoming troops feel welcome.

4. Coordinate with pastors where service personnel are attending. Discuss plans for involving them in church activities and meeting special needs of troops.

5. Visit and get acquainted with officers and chaplains having to deal with Adventist personnel.

6. Develop plans for retreats and recreational activities.

7. Work up programs that could be presented at churches and Missionary Volunteer Societies.

We had to be creative and innovative in coming up with approaches that might work. We had no facilities to use except our home which was a modest 3-bedroom ranch. We did manage to squeeze in 75 to 100 people on occasion for various social events.

There were many military locations within our area of responsibility including Walter Reed Army Hospital, Fort Myer, Quantico, Fort Meade, Bethesda Naval Hospital, and Andrews Air Force Base to name a few.

From time to time I would be called upon to help resolve problems involving Adventist servicemen within the bounds of the Columbia Union. I recall driving as far as Pennsylvania, and several times to the Norfolk, Virginia region.

By far the largest segment of our troops were in the Whitecoat unit. There were usually 150 to 200 Adventist men on the roster at any given time.

These men were divided between Fort Detrick in Frederick, Maryland and the Walter Reed Annex at Forest Glen, Maryland.

When I was a boy living in Takoma Park, the Forest Glen facility was an exclusive private girls' school, but during World

War II it was taken over by the Army and became known as Walter Reed Annex.

With this history, most of the buildings did not look like a military post. They were old and a bit rickety, but rather charming in a hilly wooded setting with a stream flowing by.

The Whitecoat unit maintained an orderly room there, and the men assigned to jobs at the annex and at the main Walter Reed Hospital were billeted there.

The larger number were assigned at Fort Detrick in Frederick where the headquarters of the unit were located. This is where the research was done, and where most of the jobs the men were assigned to from day to day took place.

In the earlier days, the men were billeted in a typical old-style wooden barracks. In the late sixties, new modern brick buildings were erected and the housing was more spacious and comfortable.

Married couples found small apartments in Frederick, or in the Takoma Park area. Usually the wives would find work in the community to help make ends meet.

Early on, the projects or studies in which volunteers allowed themselves to be exposed to infectious agents were conducted in wood barracks-type buildings which were constructed in such a way that there was a recreational courtyard where the men could play volleyball or get some fresh air. There was also an indoor recreational room or day room where they took their meals, visited, or watched television. As I remember, there was a pool table, ping pong table, and a collection of books.

As their chaplain, I was allowed to visit and conduct services, but I had to wear a hospital gown and mask, not to protect me, but to prevent my exposing them to any germs or viruses from the outside.

The projects varied as to what infectious agent was used, or what the purpose of the study might be. I remember one study where the objective was to determine what changes occur when healthy persons are confined to bed rest for weeks. No virus or bacteria was involved.

It was my observation that although some participants became uncomfortably ill with fever and aches comparable to a bad case of the flu, there were always controls who received placebo dosages and did not become sick at all.

There were also those who served out their military obligation in the Whitecoat unit and were never called upon to participate in any projects.

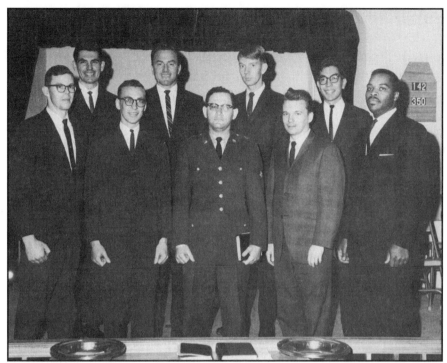

Chaplain Tom Green (back row—2nd from the left) with a group of Whitecoats at a worship service.

Of course, those who were asked to volunteer for projects always had the option to refuse. If a person continued to turn down projects without good cause, however, it would be seen by the unit as bad faith regarding his original commitment when he was selected, but he would in no instance be compelled to participate against his will.

I have talked to one or two veterans of the Whitecoat unit who feel their health has been adversely effected by being infected in these biological studies. I have heard there may be others.

My personal experience is that most Whitecoat veterans say they feel fortunate to have been selected to serve their military time in the Whitecoat unit.

In the mid-sixties I was asked to write an article about Operation Whitecoat for publication in _For God and Country_, the quarterly paper put out by the National Service Organization for distribution to Adventist military people.

The article was later put into pamphlet form, and since it sets forth my view of the unit at that time in a rather succinct way I have opted to include it here.

PROJECT WHITECOAT

1. *What is Project Whitecoat?*

Project Whitecoat is the name given to a research program conducted by the U.S. Army Medical Unit, Fort Detrick, Maryland. Participants in this project are Seventh-day Adventist soldiers who volunteer specifically for this duty. They take part in studies aimed at developing medical protective measures against disease producing organisms which might be disseminated by an enemy in the event biological warfare (germ warfare) is ever used against this country.

2. *Why are Seventh-day Adventists invited to volunteer for this unit?*

Although much of the research performed in the U.S. Army Medical Unit involves laboratory animals, some aspects of the work require human volunteers. These volunteers must be men in good health who are motivated to hazard some risk for a humanitarian cause. For purposes of research, the doctors prefer a group with as much similarity of background as possible. The volunteers must possess a good education and a variety of skills in order to fill the various jobs necessary in the operation of the unit.

In the early days of its organization, someone struck upon the idea of seeking volunteers from among the Seventh-day Adventist basic trainees at Fort Sam Houston, Texas, this being the largest single group of 1–A–0 soldiers. In this one location, men could be found who would be likely to meet the necessary qualifications. Through the years the plan has proved successful.

Not only has it been convenient for the medical unit to recruit their volunteers from a single place, but the officers have been pleased with the high level of performance and a minimum of disciplinary problems among the Seventh-day Adventist men.

3. *Who selects the volunteers?*

Once in the Spring and once in the Fall, the Commanding Officer of the medical unit and his executive officer travel to Fort Sam Houston where they extend the opportunity to volunteer to all Seventh-day Adventist soldiers in the training center there.

There are always more who volunteer than they can accept, so they endeavor to choose the men who have the skills to fill the necessary jobs, and who appear to be psychologically and emotionally equipped to fit smoothly into the unit.

They may consult the chaplain or the church representatives concerning their opinions or recommendations in certain cases, but the selection is made by the unit commander and his assistant.

4. *Does the Seventh-day Adventist Church encourage it's men to volunteer for this kind of service?*

The Army took care before instituting their plan to inquire of the church if the proposed type of volunteer service would conflict with the tenants of the Seventh-day Adventist faith. After due consideration, our church leaders replied, in substance, that for a man to volunteer to be made sick so that other people might be made well is fully consistent with Christian principles.

Since that time, the director of the National Service Organization has accompanied the officers of the Whitecoat unit on their semi-annual recruiting trips to Fort Sam Houston. His purpose is not to recruit, but to reassure the men of our denominational approval of this type of service. Whether a man volunteers for Whitecoat service must be entirely his own decision.

5. *Are there special compensations offered for those who volunteer?*

There are no special compensations offered for those who volunteer to serve in Whitecoat. It is commendable for a man to be willing to face risk in order to render a special service, but he should look for no special favors in return.

6. *Do the men spend their whole Army service period being made sick?*

No.... A volunteer will probably not be involved in more than one or two major research projects. This varies considerably. He may participate in a number of shorter projects. The rest of the time he will be assigned to a more conventional task. A number of the men work in biological, chemical, or other types of laboratories. Some are assigned as clerks, hospital specialists, animal handlers, or other jobs in keeping with their professional or technical skills.

7. Do the volunteers live and work in Washington, D. C. ?

Nearly half of the volunteers are assigned duty at the Walter Reed Army Medical Center in Washington, and live in the Walter Reed Annex in nearby Forest Glen, Maryland. The majority, however, live and work at Fort Detrick in Frederick, Maryland, which is about 50 miles north of Washington.

8. Are there advantages for me if I volunteer?

As mentioned before, there are no special compensations for this type of service, but some men consider it an advantage to know *where* they will be assigned. The Whitecoat volunteer knows he will be near Washington.

There is also a greater variety of job opportunities in Whitecoat than the medical soldier who has been drafted would find in most assignments.

The Whitecoat volunteer is also assured he will not suffer the loneliness of being isolated from others of his faith. He will be near a Seventh-day Adventist college (Columbia Union College), and there are a number of Seventh-day Adventist churches nearby. Washington is, of course, the world headquarters of the Seventh-day Adventist Church. Plans have been initiated for the establishment of a denominationally operated servicemen's center in a beautiful park-like setting near Columbia Union College in Takoma Park. This will be operation in 1967.

9. Are there disadvantages in volunteering for Whitecoat?

Many of the men who have served in Whitecoat were asked, "If you had it to do over again, would you still volunteer?" The vast majority reply that they would. Negative replies include the following comments:

1. "I've missed my opportunity to go overseas."

2. "I've not been happy in my job," or "I didn't get along well with so and so."

A certain amount of this is to be expected in any assignment.

3. "My buddy didn't volunteer and he made Spec. 5."

Promotions in the unit are as good or better than in most areas, but there are no slots for volunteers above Spec. 4.

4. "I shouldn't have risked my health."

Over 1,000 Seventh-day Adventists have participated in Project Whitecoat. Of this number less than one-half dozen have felt that such participation had affected their health. Very careful medical examination of this small group of individuals has shown no definite relationship between their subsequent complaints and their participation in this program. Most feel they have benefitted by the very thorough physical examinations they have undergone upon arrival in the unit. In a few individuals these examinations have disclosed previously unknown health problems. Needless to say, these problems received appropriate medical attention and persons with such problems have been excluded from participation in any project which might be harmful to them.

10. *Do you think it is a good idea for our men to be grouped together in a single unit? Wouldn't they do better spiritually if they were scattered?*

I include this last question because it is asked of me so frequently in one form or another. Let me say first, that we as a church have nothing to say about where soldiers of our faith are assigned. This is determined solely and entirely by the Army. As the centurion said to Jesus, "I am a man under authority, having soldiers under me: and I say to this man, Go, and he goeth; and to another, Come, and he cometh."

The Army has decided that these soldiers from Seventh-day Adventist backgrounds have a distinct service to render to their country. It is their decision to gather them in a certain unit to perform a given task.

So the key question is not whether it is a good idea for the spiritual well-being of these men for them to be grouped together in one spot. Since the Army has chosen to do this, and has brought them to the very headquarters of our church, the question is rather what can we do to influence their lives for good at this sensitive and significant time in their development. This is the reason a civilian chaplain has been appointed here, and why plans for a Servicemen's Center are being developed.

Many are concerned about the public image of our church that is projected by an Army unit that is so predominately Seventh-day Adventist. Some of these men are mature Christians and are living lives that are a real credit to their church. Others have never developed a meaningful Christian faith of their own, and project a poor image of the church whose name they bear.

We are concerned to preserve the fair name of the church, but we are even more concerned to help these young men from Adventist families to find a vital faith in Christ for themselves. We will probably have a better opportunity to do it here, with proper facilities, then if they were sent elsewhere.

—Thomas Green, Civilian Chaplain
Washington, D.C. area

In my endeavors to minister to the Whitecoat troops, I received the finest cooperation from the officers and non-commissioned officers in charge of the unit. I was given free access to visit the men either in the barracks or on the job. I tried to respect the privacy of the men and not intrude upon them, and yet to visit on a regular basis to be available to them.

As stated elsewhere, in order to be selected to be in Whitecoat a man had to be 1 –A–0 and had to declare his church preference to be Seventh-day Adventist. At that particular time in their lives, however, there was a great variance among them regarding practice of Adventist lifestyle and adherence to church standards.

Some were in a rebellious stage, reacting to the stricter limits of Adventist campus life which they had recently experienced. We were also seeing a reflection of the mood of the general society in challenging the practices of the establishment during the Vietnam war years.

Of course, a goodly number were secure in their faith commitment and lived exemplary lives in the military setting as measured by church standards.

I felt it was not in the interest of the men or the church to bring a judgmental presence into the setting in which they lived. I desired to be a representative of the church who could convey love and acceptance; to be a person who was seen as interested in them and their well being.

I was told by Colonel Crozier, the commander, and others of the officers of the unit, of the high regard and respect they had for the Adventist soldiers. The disciplinary problems were negligible. They were reliable and responsible in their work, and they brought a high level of education, and a variety of skill to the unit.

The Army was more than pleased with the recruiting arrangement that had been worked out back in the fifties, and the troops were generally equally pleased to be able to serve their military obligation in this setting. They were warned there were risks in volunteering to be involved in experimental research, but they were nowhere near the level of risk involved for those who were serving their duty in Viet Nam.

The word had gotten around the Adventist community that to be selected for Operation Whitecoat was choice duty. From time to time I would get telephone calls inquiring if I knew when the officers would be coming to Fort Sam for the selection so they could try to be there at that time hopefully to be chosen. There were usually more volunteers than there were openings, so at every selection there were some who were disappointed.

We had soldiers from every part of the country come to Whitecoat, but it seemed the greatest numbers came from California, Oregon, and Washington State. In some locations out there, it appears there is a higher percentage of Adventists to the general population making for a larger number of Adventists to be drafted from those locales. We became acquainted with a great number of Adventist young people in those days from many places, and in the ensuing years, it seems, we have run across Whitecoat veterans just about everywhere we go.

My mind turns to the development of various activities and services we tried through the years to help meet the needs of the troops.

First, I would like to give credit to the pastors and members of the Frederick Seventh-day Adventist Church. With Fort Detrick nearby, a number of servicemen and their wives attended services at the Frederick church and became involved in local church activities. The church never failed to make them feel welcome, and to extend the facilities of the church for special activities.

I remember one group of servicemen planned and conducted a series of evangelistic meetings in the old Frederick church. When the church built a new school with a fine gymnasium, they allowed us the use of the gym one night a week for volleyball, which became a favorite activity for some of the GIs.

When the new Frederick church was built, some of the troops helped with the construction. I recall joining with them in nailing roof shingles. There was a section included which was to serve as a small servicemen's center.

As Chaplain Mole mentioned in his dedication, Dr. and Mrs. Frank Damazo took the lead through the years in Frederick in fostering servicemen's activities. He and his brother Ray opened their adjoining homes and yards to us for what became a favorite annual event. It was an outdoor party on a western theme complete with horses, western music, and chuck wagon food.

After trying many types of activities there were certain events that were popular enough to repeat every year. We sponsored retreats at the youth camps. We had several at the Chesapeake Conference youth camp at Mt. Aetna, but the most popular location seemed to be the Potomac Conference site at Hidden Valley in Montebello, Virginia.

My wife continually amazed me at her ability to take on the task of feeding 100 to 150 people for an entire weekend. We usually had a special speaker who would appeal to the young adults such as Ed Peterson, from the Columbia Union or Bob Schwindt from the college.

Other favorite repeat activities were the banquets at the Peter Pan Restaurant near Frederick, the all-day gatherings at the Review & Herald chapel, or the Sanitarium chapel and gym.

Memorable, but limited as far as numbers, were the camping outings to New England at the turning of the leaves; the outer banks of North Carolina, and the canoe trip to Algonquin Provincial Park in Canada. There was also the trip to the Youth Congress held in Atlantic City in the mid-sixties. The servicemen were given a special part in the pageantry.

In the early years when we had no facilities of our own, we had to beg and plead with some of our established Adventist institutions in Takoma Park for space.

For the single servicemen, Columbia Union College offered a great attraction. The weekend programs planned for the students were also of some interest to the troops, but the most important element, simply put, is that's where the girls were.

My wife taught nursing at the college during those years. Her students were mostly female. As a result, many of her girls attended our social events and met my boys. There are quite a number of married couples across the country who first met under these fortuitous circumstances.

Since Fort Detrick was about 50 miles from Takoma Park, we thought it would be well if some reasonably priced lodging could be found near the college.

The school had recently completed the new boys' dormitory and classroom facility called Morrison Hall. As a result, the old wooden dormitory, North Hall, had been closed. Dr. Winton Beaven was college president at the time, and he was open-thinking enough to see wisdom in re-opening North Hall on weekends to accommodate the troops. I believe this was not only a compassionate decision on the part of the school, but very likely influenced some of the men to enroll at Columbia Union College when they returned to school after completing their military obligation.

The Washington Sanitarium several times allowed us the use of their chapel and gymnasium for all-day Sabbath meetings and Saturday night socials. After a time, it became clear that our gatherings were attracting a lot of people and the Sanitarium administrators realized it was costing them parking spaces which they needed for patients and visitors. Also the soldiers were becoming familiar with the facility, and were feeling comfortable relaxing in the Sanitarium lounges. We were informed regretfully that we would no longer be welcome to use their facilities.

We had some gatherings at the Review and Herald Chapel, and at the old General Conference building. We were grateful for help extended by the various Church facilities, but it was awkward always having to beg and borrow.

THE WASHINGTON SERVICEMEN'S CENTER

One of the methods we tried at the beginning was organizing servicemen's committees to explore needs, and plan activities. They even produced a newsletter that was sent out for a time.

One proposal that came out of those committees was the need for a servicemen's center in Takoma Park. Even after the committees ceased to function, when groups of soldiers would sit around discussing needs and hopes, the matter of a Servicemen's Center would arise.

They talked about the ideal location—within walking distance of the college. They talked about what it should look like—noninstitutional, warm and inviting. They talked about the services it should provide, and the allocation of space for these purposes. They definitely felt the function should be clearly defined first, and the form should follow.

Bill King, one of the soldiers stationed at Walter Reed, had studied architecture in civilian life, and he was so interested he came up with a very fine preliminary floor plan and elevation. This is not the plan that was ultimately built, but it was a beginning and helped to stir interest in the project.

I still have a long list of signatures prepared by the soldiers requesting a facility be established near Columbia Union College where they could stay on weekends. In our collective dream, we spoke of the ideal location being a "retreat-like setting" which would help provide a restful, non-military atmosphere.

Having grown up in Takoma Park, I remembered some denominationally owned property bordering Long Branch park. I had played there as a teenager.

It had once been part of the parcel designated for Potomac University, before the decision was made to establish the University at the Emmanual Missionary College campus in Michigan. The property lay behind the athletic fields of Takoma Academy. It was rich with trees, commanded a beautiful view of the park, and Long Branch Creek, and was only five blocks from the college.

Elder Ted Lucas was secretary (director) of the Missionary Volunteer (youth) department of the General Conference of which the National Service Organization was a part. In June of 1965 he wrote to me, "There is nothing that seems a greater need to me in the area of the National Service Organization than a servicemen's center here in Washington, D.C. I have said to the men who are in responsible positions of the General Conference that this is the greatest need in the world for our National Service Organization at the moment."

He was a great source of encouragement to me. He said even though it seemed things were moving slowly, he felt sure our hopes for a servicemen's center in Washington area would materialize. I remember one day running into Elder Lucas in the lobby of the Washington Sanitarium. I asked him if he had a few minutes to look at a piece of property with me, and he agreed. I cherish the memory

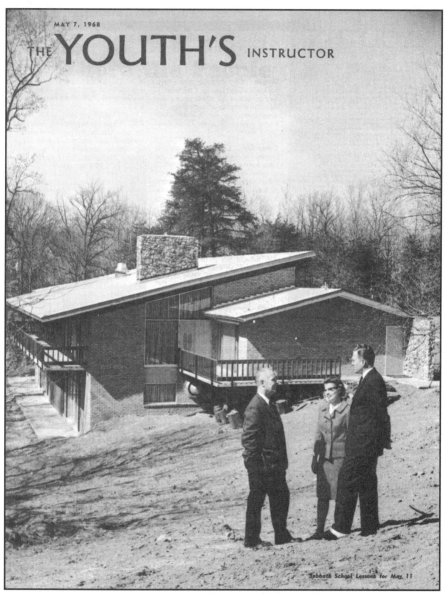

Servicemen's Center in Takoma Park, MD.

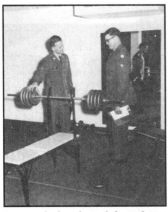

SP4 Paul Chambers, left, and SP4 Charles Randall inspect some of the recreation facilities.

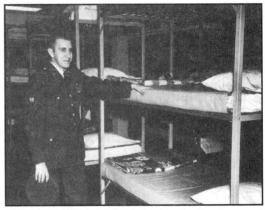

SP4 George Francis stands in the sixty-bunk ground floor of the center.

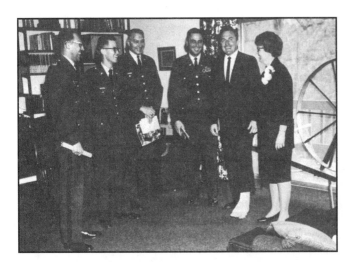

Hosts to those visiting were Thomas A. Green and wife, Priscilla. In uniform, from left, stand Col. William Beisel, SP4 Ron Bechtel, 1st Sgt. George Redinger, Lt. Col. Orlyn Oestereich.

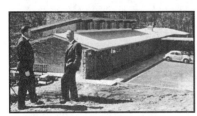

Thomas Green and Clark Smith converse, with the Washington Servicemen's Center in the background.

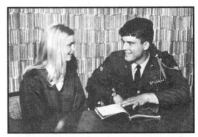

A brief tete-a-tete is enjoyed by Sarah Blackburn and Glenn Stimpson, who recently returned from Vietnam.

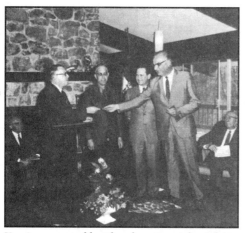

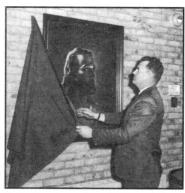

G.D. Bras unveils gift picture from Potomac Conference

Key is presented by Theodore Carcich, right to Theodore Lucas, left with Enos Levy, builder, and Richard Hart, architect, looking on.

Chief of Chaplains Maj. Gen. Francis L. Sampson, gives his address. Those seated left to right are, C. Smith, T. Lucas, Col. George T. Casey, Robert H. Pierson, T. Carcich, and O.A. Blake.

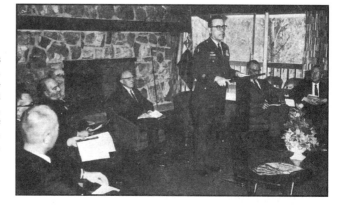

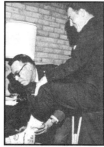

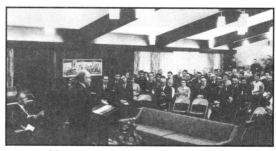

Maj. Gen. Francis L. Sampson, autographs Elder Thomas Green's New Cast.

Elder Pierson speaks in the large lounge.

of walking over the beautiful site with that good man. It seemed we shared a vision of what could be. The setting could not have been more ideal for our proposed purpose.

Other possibilities were explored, but in time this did become the site that was chosen. It was at that time the property of the Potomac Conference, though it previously had been owned by the General Conference back in Potomac University days. The Potomac Conference agreed to lease the land back to the General Conference for the purpose of building a servicemen's center with the proviso that should the building ever cease to be used for that function, the entire property would revert to the Potomac Conference.

A key figure in making the dream of a servicemen's center become a reality was Elder Neal Wilson, while serving as president of the North American division. It was Elder Wilson who presented the proposal to the Fall Council and obtained an initial appropriation of $160,000 so that building plans could go forward.

It must have been the 1963 Fall Council which appropriated the funds because in early 1964 Elder 0. A. Blake, Elder Ed Peterson, and I were appointed as an investigating committee regarding the location of the center in Takoma Park.

Elder Peterson was another source of great encouragement in my work. He was very much in touch with the needs of the servicemen, and the problems associated with trying to coordinate spiritual and social activities for them. Eventually, his own son, Bob, would be drafted into the Army and become one of the Whitecoat soldiers.

In a letter to the General Conference officers in May of 1964, Elder Peterson estimated the number of SDA servicemen in the Washington area would increase to 300 and would continue at that level for the foreseeable future. It was impossible for any of us to anticipate at that time the military draft would end only eight years later, and drastically alter the situation.

With funds made available by the General Conference, we plunged ahead to help the dream of a servicemen's center in Takoma Park become a reality.

An operating board for the yet-to-be-built center was formed in January 1966 with Elder Lucas as chairman and representatives from the General Conference, the Columbia Union, and Potomac Conference. A building committee was also named which was chaired by Elder Ted Carcich and had strong representation from the Missionary Volunteer Department including the director of the National Service Organization, Elder Clark Smith, and his associate Elder Charles Martin. These men were heavily involved in carrying forward plans for construction and operation of the center.

Another key person from the Missionary Volunteer staff was Elder Lawrence Nelson who was gifted with an artistic sense and contributed greatly toward selection of furnishings and appointments to make the interior of the building attractive and in good taste.

We were fortunate to have the services of a young Adventist architect from Rhodesia (Zimbabwe) to design the building. His name was Richard "Buddy" Hart and he took a deep personal interest in the project from the beginning. I appreciated the fact that he took time to listen carefully to the description of needs we had thought about so long, and the mood we felt the structure should convey. He made a contribution by greatly reducing his fee, and reduced costs by incorporating in the plan materials and construction techniques that were economical, yet produced a rich appearance. He also recommended to us an Adventist builder by the name of Enos Levy who did an excellent job for us in construction.

The final product was everything we had asked for, and more attractive than we had hoped.

Constructed of brick and stone accented with heavy wooden beams it reminded some of an attractive ski lodge. The scenic location overlooking the park and stream helped make the facility very inviting.

The main floor featured a very large lounge (60' x 30') with a massive stone fireplace and exposed wooden beams. There were sliding glass doors leading out to a large balcony overlooking the beautiful scene below.

Adjoining the lounge was a well equipped kitchen with snack bar, and a dining area large enough for 3 or 4 tables. There was a small library room which afforded a quiet area for reading and writing, and served well as a place for small committee meetings.

The first floor also included two offices, and an apartment for the Chaplain and his family. This was to afford live-in supervision for the facility.

The lower level had a barracks-like sleeping area which could accommodate 60 men, a recreation room, and a small apartment for a couple who could assist in the operation. There were also 4 motel-like guest rooms to accommodate married couples, or ladies in military service. Because of the sloping lot, the lower level was above ground and exited to the grass area surrounded by lovely trees in the back.

The opening ceremony for the new Servicemen's Center was held February 28, 1968. Guest speakers were Major General Francis Sampson, Chief of Chaplains of the U.S. Army and Robert H. Pierson, President of the General Conference of Seventh-day Adventists.

There were many present that day to celebrate the fulfillment of a dream, made possible by the sacrificial efforts of a great number of people. Church leaders, military officers and enlisted men, planners, architect and builders, and volunteers who donated countless hours were there. There was one soldier, Bob Acquistapace, who gave literally hundreds of hours of labor through the entire project. Numbers of others joined with me to do all of the painting. Dr. Arvil Bunch, an Adventist civilian who was director of Army Educational Services, and Colonel Sanford Graves who was stationed at the Pentagon, both donned their paint clothes on several occasions to pitch in and help.

The spirit of helpfulness continued as we began to operate the facility. One GI, who was a whiz with electronics, designed and installed a much needed sound system. This was his gift to the center. Others pitched in to help with the landscaping, and to clean up the woods. One soldier with experience in lumbering took down a huge tree that was dangerously close to the building.

On the first Sabbath the facility was open, very early the doorbell rang. When my wife went to answer she found three men. One had blood running down his face from a lacerated scalp, the second was holding a bayonet in one hand and a large rock in the other, and the third was holding a gun.

They shouted to her to please call the police. The man with the bloody face had just held up a nearby service station by pressing the bayonet into the stomach of the mechanic on duty. After taking all the money in the cash register he ran across the street to change into some clothes he had hidden behind the Book and Bible House. The mechanic got a gun and gave chase, joined by an off-duty soldier who had been working on his car at the station. The soldier was younger, and caught up with the robber halfway across the athletic field behind Takoma Academy. He picked up a rock and hit the robber over the head knocking him down and causing the laceration. They took the robber's bayonet, and directed him at gun point to the nearest source of help which happened to be the new servicemen's center.

This was a rather rude awakening for us. Our retreat-like setting was not free from the hazards of the real world. It was then we began to explore security measures we might take. It seemed providential that later that same week, Ron, one of our former soldiers, came to the center to ask if we knew anyone who would like to have a German Shepherd dog.

He was a fine animal, only a year old with a gentle nature, but who had demonstrated his courage in driving off two muggers who had tried to attack Ron one evening while he was jogging. They hadn't noticed the dog who was not on a leash, and off to the side a bit. I guess they thought Ron would be easy prey, but suddenly the dog was on them and they made a hasty exit. As we heard the story my wife and I both had a single thought. We asked if we could see him. Ron said, "Of course, he's right out in the car." Ron hated to part with him, but he was moving to an apartment where pets were not permitted.

The dog's name was Fitz. He was all we could have hoped for. He was gentle and friendly, but at the same time, very strong and courageous.

His favorite game was chasing a flashlight beam. The fellows loved to play the game with him. He would chase the spot of light all around, but if you shined the beam on your shoe, he would stop and stare at it until the light moved off the foot and he would begin the chase again.

One night I had to go down into Washington. Priscilla asked me to take Fitz along saying she would feel safer if he were with me. We came to an intersection where a policeman was directing traffic with a flashlight. Fitz was sure the policeman wanted to play, and the flashlight beam was for his benefit.

Unknowingly, we had seen Fitz before. His picture was featured on the front cover of the Junior Guide magazine. I had admired the picture, not knowing he would one day be our dog.

Fitz became a favorite at the Center and he helped us feel more secure. We had to deal with many types of people in our work there. He was a warm furry friend to our G.I. guests, but a deterrent to strangers who might have mischief in mind.

Eight years later his kidneys failed. I held him in my arms while the veterinarian administered the fatal injection that released him from the anguish of a slower dying process. I wept unashamedly as the vet left me quietly alone with him. I felt I had lost a good friend, as well as one who had helped me in a special ministry at a special time. His name never appeared in the obituaries of denominational workers in the Review and Herald, but he had made the front cover of Junior Guide.

It may be well to describe the operation of the Washington Servicemen's Center during its brief history. In the event universal military service should return, it could be the church will resort once again to this type of facility to meet the needs of its youth.

The Washington Servicemen's Center was a fine facility, and the only one we had the advantage of designing and constructing specifically for its intended use. The others in San Antonio, Tacoma, Washington, Seoul, and Frankfurt were converted from private homes.

The center bore the test of time and use. Even after years of service, we were convinced the plan had been well thought out, and provided the right allocation of space within our cost constraints. It could well serve as a model for future facilities if the need should arise again.

Getting the operation underway was a significant challenge. There were many matters needing attention in finishing the building, and furnishing it.

The physical plant was 12,000 square feet with an acre of grounds. We needed to obtain tools and equipment for the cleaning and maintenance of the building and grounds, as well as kitchen and office supplies and equipment so we could perform our functions.

We had some concepts in the planning stages regarding staffing, but these had to be refined as we got underway. It was to be a family operation. I was to be the director of the facility, and my wife, Priscilla, was to be the secretary and treasurer. She resigned her position as nursing instructor at Columbia Union College, and we sold our home and moved into the apartment provided on the main floor. The apartment downstairs was designed to house a couple who could help with the operation and maintenance in exchange for free rent.

Time demonstrated that even though we all pitched in to help, cleaning and maintenance required hiring additional people. Ultimately, the plan that worked best was carefully selecting a serviceman and wife to occupy the apartment. We looked for qualities such as maturity, demonstration of Christian values, and the capacity to relate well to guests. All of the couples who served had good educational backgrounds.

In exchange for free lodging they agreed to be on duty two nights per week and every other weekend. This meant answering the phone, receiving guests, opening and locking up the building, assisting the men with their needs, and dealing with problems and emergencies as they arose.

I remember each of the couples with fondness and I would like to honor their service by listing their names in the order in which they served.

1. Clifford and Diana Bartholomew

2. Tommy and Ina McFarland

3. Don and Kathy Stiles

4. Larry and Jane Dodds

5. Clifford and Karen Ingersoll

I remember, too, the young people who worked in the maintenance responsibilities. It was important that the building and grounds should be clean and neat, but it was equally important that those we employed should relate well to the guests. Craig Hufnagle, Richard Truitt, Alfred Watson, Larry Carter, and JoAnne Ellis were especially helpful. We would supplement with occasional help from servicemen or ex-servicemen who came to us and were short of money. We were able to extend financial help to them in this way.

Operating the servicemen's center was a 24-hour seven-day-a-week job. We became an extended family for the troops far from home. In some ways I became a father figure, and Priscilla a mother figure. My mother, who often came to help out, was called grandma by everyone, and my children were like siblings to the young men and women.

Perhaps an effective way to describe the operation at the center is to quote from a report I submitted to the National Service Organization in January of 1973.

"Our usage is increased. We have a lot of new men coming to the Whitecoat program and more are being assigned to the Washington area again."

"This weekend we provided lodging for 57 people which is nearly maximum. The hospitality dinner at Sligo Church is not operating temporarily and the college dining room was closed, so we provided Sabbath dinner in addition to the normal breakfast fare. We also served chili on Friday night."

"Through the holiday season we provided lodging for over 100 different people, though not all at the same time. We had about 45 over New Year's weekend though not so many over Christmas. Many of the men who normally would come here had Christmas leave."

"We had a Christmas party on Saturday night preceding Christmas with about 60 present. On Christmas eve we had a less structured event with 30 present. At Christmas dinner we had 15 guests. We had approximately 80 present at our New Year's celebration. We ushered in the New Year with an invitation for a new commitment to Christ."

"The various functions held here during November and December include two meetings of the Adventist Forum, the General Conference Ladies Auxiliary with Dr. Hyde speaking on Glossolalia, Sligo Church potluck, Single girls' party, Thanksgiving dinner, Missionary Volunteer Council, Ski Club, and Publishing Department meeting."

Let me insert here that we permitted various meetings and functions to be held at the Center with the provision they must be compatible with the interests of the servicemen, and they be permitted to participate if they should choose. One week we had a Valentine's party plus a vegetarian banquet by the Civitan Club, and another banquet of Spanish food put on by the Spanish Adventist Church.

We cooperated in a roller skating function each Saturday night at a local rink which was reserved exclusively for Adventists. We also kept the men informed of other activities in the Takoma park area that might be of interest to them.

The 1973 report continues, "Back to a description of current duties, a great deal of time is spent in meeting the needs of the people who come here. People require time. We try to thoroughly orient each new man to the facility, and make him feel at home. We try to convey a concept of each man maintaining his own area and cleaning up his own mess in the kitchen. They are pretty good, but it takes continual reinforcing and picking up after."

"We spend a lot of time talking with the men. We help them with their emergencies like being stranded at the airport or bus station, or a car that won't start in some very inconvenient location. We try to evaluate these requests as to whether it is something the man could handle himself or something with which he really needs help. Frequently the men just want to be reassured of our interest in them, but many hours are spent counseling about significant problems."

"A great deal of time is spent handling telephone traffic and doorbells. When we have as many people as we do staying in a facility like this, life seems a constant series of interruptions of this kind. We get a surprising number of calls from people who interpret Washington Servicemen's Center as Adventist Information Center."

"A significant amount of time is spent planning and carrying out social activities for the men. Our next major event is a banquet at the Peter Pan restaurant on January 23."

"We conduct two major retreats each year in the Spring and Fall usually at the Blue Ridge Youth Camp in Virginia. Attendance is usually 75 to 100."

"Priscilla and I have been in this work for 11 years now. We have operated the Servicemen's Center for five. The first six years were interesting, but frustrating without adequate facilities. The last five have been even more interesting, and it has been wonderful to be able to offer the hospitality of this excellent facility."

"Life in the center is unique. We have surrendered our privacy, but we have touched many lives. It is like living in a beehive where interruptions are the rule rather than the exception. Our work requires us to be flexible, and adaptable. It involves much "waiting on tables" and many humble tasks. The needs of the men dictate our schedules and frequently turn night into day. Our holidays belong to the men. Our meals are frequently shared with them, and are usually interrupted by them."

"Life here has had its effects on our family life, some good, some bad. Family communication is difficult. An uninterrupted family conversation is a rare luxury. Coverage of the center often interferes with Priscilla and me doing things together. But we have our compensations. We may be confined, but never bored. And there are times when things ease up and we can slip away to catch up with ourselves."

"Things appear to be uncertain as to the future of our NSO work and the continued operation of the Servicemen's Center . . . I assume that in the next couple of years something may happen to require a change."

"Let me say I have appreciated the opportunity to be in this specialized work. Whatever happens in the future, I am thankful for this experience which has been ours—to work with you and Charles and others in the department; to share experiences with the other Chaplains and feel the warmth of their fellowship though spread around the world in our common task."

"Many of the men and women we have ministered to have seemed like sons and daughters to us. The number must be in the thousands, with hundreds we have come to know well."

The words of that report written nearly 20 years ago on the scene probably capture the story better than my fading memory can serve to do. It was only one and one-half years later the Center did indeed close. As the agreement with the Potomac Conference had stated, should the facility cease to be used as a servicemen's center it would revert to the conference. It has been used as a Takoma Park office for the Potomac Conference since that time.

I received an invitation to serve as Chaplain at Porter Memorial Hospital in Denver, Colorado beginning in June 1974 where I continued my ministry until retirement in January of 1990.

As I reflect back on my years of Chaplaincy I consider it was a wonderful privilege and opportunity to perform a needed service. The people I met both in military and hospital settings taught me valuable lessons about life, and about what really matters most.

The hours were long and often the demands were overwhelming.

I am thankful for my wife, Priscilla, who had an amazing ability to adapt to the special stresses of our work. I don't know many women who could have followed Christ's example so literally in feeding the 5,000. She pursued our mutual task with energy, and willingly set aside personal interests for the good of those we served.

Since our troops came to us from all parts of the country, it has afforded us special pleasure to meet them again just about everywhere we go. We rejoice in their successes, and feel sorrow when we hear of their pain. In some cases we meet the children of couples we introduced many years ago.

Let me close by quoting from a letter I once wrote to Elder Ted Lucas.

"Several times this week I have heard the comment, 'There is no other church in the world that takes such good care of its servicemen.' That is true, and I'm glad to be a part of it."

Priscilla and I are both still glad to have been a part of that very special caring ministry.

Postscript

I struggled with the matter of including names of servicemen we ministered to and who ministered to us in return. I opted not to try to use many names for reasons of space limitations, and the fear that while I remember some vividly, I would forget others just as important. To all our military friends from those days in the 60's and early 70's, our fondest greetings wherever you are. It was good to know you, and thank you for enriching us as our lives touched briefly in a special time and place.

Chaplain and Mrs. Tom Green

Tom was certified in 1976 as a Fellow in the College of Chaplains of the American Protestant Hospital Association.

He continued to serve as a Chaplain at Porter Memorial Hospital in Denver until his retirement in January of 1990.

He and his wife Priscilla reside in the beautiful valley of Ken Caryl in Littleton, Colorado conveniently near their children.

POSTSCRIPT

A vigorous program of biomedical research at USAMRIID continues today. In some ways, the threat posed by infectious disease, both natural and manmade, is greater today than ever. Even the Whitecoat volunteers continue to make contributions more than 25 years after the end of the program.

A new program is underway at USAMRIID to perform a health assessment of former Whitecoat participants. Lieutenant Colonel Phillip Pittman, Deputy Chief of the Medical Division is spearheading a program designed to study the effects of multiple vaccinations on long term health. With the rapidly increasing immunization requirements of U.S. servicemen and women, this area of inquiry is gaining importance.

Interested Operation Whitecoat participants should contact:

LTC Phillip Pittman, MC, USA
USAMRIID
1425 Porter Street
Fort Detrick, MD 21702–5011

Your participation would provide very valuable data and help to insure the health and welfare of our young men and women in uniform.

As previously mentioned, human research continues at USAMRIID. Excerpts from a letter sent to Dr. Damazo by the chairman of the Human Use and Ethics committee reads:

24 April 1998

The present program at USAMRIID for research involving human subjects has numerous links to the groundwork laid by the U.S. Army Medical Unit and Project Whitecoat...copies of procedures currently in operation at USAMRIID illustrate this fact.

Medical Research Volunteer Subjects (MRVS) are recruited semi-annually from the 91B school at Fort Sam Houston, Texas using procedures that are virtually identical to those of Project Whitecoat.

When I first chaired the "modern" Human Use Committee (now called the Institutional Review Board or IRB) beginning in 1975, I took for granted that the methods for recruiting the subject population were unique. It was not until I accompanied the team to report on their practices that I noted the "Acknowledgment" signed by the potential MRVS still contained the "promise of noncombatant duty" which identifies this document as related to "Whitecoat." This was 1993 and we were still "promising noncombatant duty" despite abolishment of the Draft in 1971 and the existence of an "All Volunteer Army." I was able to correct the documents for future use, but smiled introspectively about the heritage of Project Whitecoat that the Adventists had given us.

The process of review and approval of protocols has become more complex due to increased specific "rules" about review and a movement away from use of principles like the Nuremberg Code, but there are also many other requirements to document. This has resulted in more uniformity of ethical practices in military research and has made the process less dependent on the specific credentials of the individual IRB chairs.

The Human Use Committee has been successful in enforcing these principles of Informed Consent, Minimization of Risks, Protection of Rights and Welfare for over 20 years since commencing in 1975.

These documents have not been published verbatim anywhere else and if you find them useful to document my respect and continuance of the program, please feel free to include them. (Readers interested in current standards are invited to review Appendix C.)

Arthur O. Anderson, MD
COL MC
Human Use and Ethics

*****

An extremely well written article by Caree Vander Linden is reproduced with permission from the August 1997 issue of *Soldiers* magazine.

When troops are deployed, in peace time or war, they may face invisible enemies —infectious diseases—that can be as hostile as any human foe.

The U.S. Army Medical Research Institute of Infectious Diseases (USAMRIID) at Fort Detrick, MD, is working to counter this threat by developing vaccines, drugs and diagnostic tests to protect U.S. forces from diseases and biological warfare agents. About 70 USAMRIID soldiers play a special role in this mission: They are Medical Research Volunteer Subjects (MRVS), who come to USAMRIID to participate in clinical trials of new vaccines and drugs.

Corporal Mark Phillips, a former MRVS, said he took a lot of kidding from fellow soldiers at Fort Sam Houston, Texas, when he decided to volunteer, but he still feels good about his decision.

"I saw it as a chance to help people," Phillips said. "Somewhere down the road, all the guys who picked on me are going to benefit from this research. What we're doing is for the good of the country."

According to Major Trinka Coster, director of clinical studies in USAMRIID's Medical Division, "Any drug that you can buy at your local pharmacy has been tested on people—in clinical trials much like these—before being approved by the U.S. Food and Drug Administration. The difference at USAMRIID is that we test drugs and vaccines to protect U.S. Troops."

While some civilians from the local community participate in USAMRIID's trials, the institute relies heavily on its in-house volunteers, most of whom are recruited from the combat medic unit at Fort Sam Houston.

Being an MRVS is typically a three-year assignment in which volunteers work in the labs and offices throughout USAMRIID, part of the U.S. Army Medical Research and Material Command (USAMRMC). While gaining firsthand experience in a research environment, they also have a number of educational opportunities.

During his stint as an MRVS, Phillips attended college and completed several Army correspondence courses. He pursued his Expert Field Medical Badge and attended Air Assault School. And he chose to participate in vaccine trials for sandfly fever, shigella and Rift Valley Fever.

"The MRVSs aren't required to participate—it's completely voluntary," Coster said. "They're only required to listen to the study protocol when it's presented and they can withdraw at any time—even if the study is already in progress."

According to Coster, vaccines and drugs tested at USAMRIID have been studied extensively in animals before human testing begins. The next step is to gauge the safety and immunity-producing effectiveness of these products in human volunteers.

"Safety trials tell us if a product has any side effects," Coster said. "Studies also show us whether a product produces an immune response to protect against disease. To assess that response, we periodically take blood samples from volunteers and measure the antibodies they've developed."

For diseases such as malaria, for which effective treatments are available, study volunteers may be "challenged" after vaccination. This exposes them to the infectious agent that causes malaria to determine whether the vaccine protects them from infection. If the vaccine fails to protect them and they show symptoms of malaria, they immediately receive proper health care with proven medications.

Diseases like anthrax, however, are too dangerous to be used in human "challenge" studies. In such cases, studies are conducted using animal models only—human volunteers are never exposed to the disease. Instead, they receive the anthrax vaccine—which is a licensed product—and have their blood tested for antibodies.

"Antibodies produced by the human volunteers are the given to anthrax-exposed animals," Coster said. "If the antibodies protect the animals from the disease, the vaccine is considered a potential success."

Depending on the length of the study, volunteers can expect to have periodic follow-up visits and blood draws. The MRVSs are monitored closely during the first 30 to 60 days of a trial, less frequently after that.

Most clinical trials are done on an outpatient basis, but some protocols require volunteers to be monitored 24 hours a day to ensure that outside factors don't influence results. These studies are conducted in USAMRIID's inpatient ward, which is equipped with private sleeping rooms, exercise equipment, a game area and lounge.

The ward is also used for inpatient trials of products developed by the Walter Reed Army Institute of Research (WRAIR) and the Naval Medical Research Institute.

"We work closely with other military organizations," said Coster. "For example, we were part of the team that developed the hepatitis A vaccine, and we've tested several vaccines and drugs developed by WRAIR—including those for dengue and malaria."

Such diseases are a major threat to U.S. forces. In the Vietnam era, infectious diseases were responsible for two-thirds of all hospital admissions. Today in Bosnia, American troops may face a number of exotic viruses, including the one that causes tick-borne encephalitis. More than 3,000 troops have been immunized against this threat, thanks to a TBE vaccine that was tested at USAMRIID.

The military is currently conducting a large-scale field trial of an oral cholera vaccine that was earlier tested at USAMRIID. If these results hold up in the field trial, the vaccine could be used not only for troops, but in the developing nations where cholera is widespread, Coster said.

While USAMRIID is primarily focused on research to protect soldiers, the institute occasionally works with private industry to test products that could benefit civilian populations as well as the military.

"We're not in the business of manufacturing products, just developing them," said Coster. "If we can tie in with industry and have them absorb some of the costs, it benefits all of us."

In addition to following the same federal regulations that govern commercial drug companies, clinical trials at USAMRIID must comply with Army regulations.

Before a study involving human volunteers can begin, it must be approved by USAMRIID's Scientific Review Committee, which reviews each proposal for scientific merit and mission relevance.

The institute's Human Use Committee then reviews the proposal to ensure it meets strict ethical standards that protect the volunteers.

If approved at this level, the proposal goes to USAMRMC and ultimately to the Office of the Surgeon General for final approval.

Colonel Arthur Anderson, who chairs the Human Use Committee, says the group doesn't hesitate to modify or reject a proposal if it doesn't adequately reduce risk or meet other criteria required by regulations.

Before participating in a study, each volunteer receives an informed consent packet that includes detailed information on the study, why it's being conducted and any possible adverse effects. After reading the material, the volunteer must sign a consent form before being allowed to participate.

Phillips, who is now stationed at the USAMRMC Office of the Secretary of the General Staff, said his symptoms were mostly minor.

"Sometimes I had diarrhea, or maybe a headache—nothing serious," he said. "Once I came down with sandfly fever, and had a 102-degree temperature. But I knew from the consent form that there was a chance I might get sick."

"They take care of us here," said Sergeant Lisa Sheridan-Cuddy, who has been an MRVS for two years. Her husband Specialist Lancer Cuddy, is also an MRVS and was recruited from the same graduating class. Both said the opportunity for continuing education motivated them to volunteer.

"One of the main reasons I came here was that I knew I'd be able to finish my college degree," Sheridan-Cuddy said. "I'm now in the process of applying to medical school."

She recalled telling other students in her Primary Leadership Development Course about life at USAMRIID.

"When they heard about it, everyone in my class wanted to come to Fort Detrick," she said. "It's a great assignment."

APPENDIXES

APPENDIX A

VITAE

BRIGADIER GENERAL WILLIAM D. TIGERTT, M.D.
UNITED STATES ARMY, RETIRED (Deceased)

William D. Tigertt was born in Wilmer, Texas on 22 May 1915. He earned his baccalaureate degree in 1937 and his medical degree in 1938 from Baylor University, Waco, Texas. Medical residencies in Medicine and Pathology continued at Baylor from 1937 to September 1940, at which time he accepted an Army Commission as a Pathologist. First assigned to the U.S. Army's Brooke General Hospital in San Antonio, Texas, he had many other exciting and demanding tours of duty.

During his military service, Doctor Tigertt held responsible roles as Commanding Officer, 26th Army Medical Laboratory in New Guinea, the Philippines, and Japan from 1944 to 1946; the 406th U.S. General Laboratory in Tokyo from 1946 to 1949; Assistant Commandant, Walter Reed Army Institute of Research from 1949 to 1956; Commanding Officer, U.S. Army Medical Institute of Research from 1949 to 1956; Director and Commandant, Walter Reed Army Institute of Research, which is now the United States Army Medical Research Institute of Infectious Diseases (USAMRIID). General Tigertt completed his military career as Commanding Officer, Madigan General Hospital, Fort Lewis, Washington in 1972.

Following retirement from the Army in 1972 he joined the faculty of the University of Maryland School of Medicine as Professor of Medicine, and Professor and Associate Chairman of the Department of Pathology. He also directed the clinical laboratories of the University Hospital.

Doctor Tigertt was editor of the *American Journal of Tropical Medicine* from 1983 to 1990. He was a Diplomate of the American Board of Pathology, and a Fellow of the American College of Physicians. Doctor Tigertt was the recipient of numerous awards and citations. These included the Bronze Star Medal, United States Army, 1945; the United States Army Commendation Medal, 1946; the Legion of Merit, 1965; the Gorgas Medal, Association of Military Surgeons, 1966; the Kober Lecturer of the Association of American Physicians, 1975; and the Joseph E. Smadel Award and Lecturer, 1990.

Brigadier General William D. Tigertt died on Sunday, 19 January 1992, in the Walter Reed Army Hospital, Washington, D.C., following a brief illness.

In spite of the heavy scientific responsibilities and positions which he held, Doctor Tigertt found time to associate, communicate and often inspire his associates in the arena of medical research. Theodore E. Woodward, M.D., a long-time scientific associate of General Tigertt, verbalized so well the respect and appreciation experienced by many of the Whitecoat participants.

"Bill Tigertt had one of the most productive scientific minds in the military service, and through his great organizational abilities was able to accomplish many important things which not only benefited the military services but the general public as well. He was a pathfinder in the field of Preventive Medicine."

COLONEL DAN CROZIER, M.D.
UNITED STATES ARMY, RETIRED

Colonel Dan Crozier was born 25 December 1914 in Matoaka, West Virginia. He completed his premedical studies at the University of West Virginia in 1935, and received his medical degree from Harvard Medical School in 1939. After a two year internship at the Methodist Hospital, Brooklyn, New York, Colonel Crozier was commissioned a First Lieutenant in the United States Army Medical Corps on 27 May 1941, and entered active duty on 7 July 1941. Promotions were received during the following years until he achieved the rank of Colonel, Medical Corps, 27 July 1959.

During World War II Colonel Crozier served in the Middle East theater in the following assignments: Attending Surgeon, U.S. Military North African Mission; Surgeon, Heliopolis Depot; Surgeon, Libyan Service Command; Surgeon, Tripoli Base Command; and Medical Inspector, Delta Service Command. Following his overseas duty he was an instructor at the Medical Field Service School at Carlisle Barracks, Pennsylvania, and later at Brooke Army Medical Center, Fort Sam Houston, Texas. During 1946 and 1947, he was detailed to the Antarctic as the Army Medical Service observer with the Byrd Expedition. Following this assignment, he was appointed Professor of Military Science and Tactics at Vanderbilt University School of Medicine, where he simultaneously completed a year of advanced studies under a Fellowship program and a year of senior residency training in internal medicine at the Oliver General Hospital, Augusta, Georgia. Colonel Crozier is certified by the American Board of Internal Medicine and holds the 'A' prefix awarded by The Surgeon General for outstanding achievement in his professional specialty.

During the Korean War, Colonel Crozier served as Chief of the Medical Service at the U.S. Army Hospital, Camp Rucker, Alabama (1950 to 1953), as the Medical Consultant to the Eighth U.S. Army in Korea (1953 to 1954), and as Chief of Medicine at the Ryukyu Army Hospital in Okinawa (1954 to 1956). In 1956 he returned to the United States to the Office of The Surgeon General in Washington, D.C., where he served as Assistant Chief Medical Consultant until 1958 when he was appointed Chief Medical Consultant. He became the Commanding Officer of the U.S. Army Medical Unit (later USAMRIID) at Fort Detrick, Frederick, Maryland, in 1961.

In addition to his primary duty as Commander, USAMRIID, Colonel Crozier served as Consultant to The Surgeon General, Department of the Army, for infectious diseases and medical defense against biological warfare; Deputy Director, Commission on Epidemiological Survey, Armed Forces Epidemiological Board; United States Representative to The Panel of Experts on Medical Aspects of Biological Operations, North Atlantic Treaty Organization; and Associate Professor of Medicine, University of Maryland.

Following retirement from active military service on 30 March 1973, Colonel Crozier became Director, Whittaker Corporation, Indonesian Hospital Project, until 1974. Since 1974 he has been a Consultant, Whittaker Corporation, Saudi Arabian Hospital Project.

During his military service he earned the following decorations and awards:

— Legion of Merit
— Army Commendation Medal with Oak Leaf Cluster
— European-African-Middle Eastern Campaign Medal
— American Defense Service Medal
— United Nations Service Medal
— Korean Service Medal
— American Campaign Medal
— World War II Victory Medal
— Antarctica Service Medal
— Gorgas Medal

Colonel Crozier has published a large number of scientific papers, is certified by the American Board of Internal Medicine, and holds an 'A' prefix rating in that specialty. He is a member of the following professional organizations: Fellow in the American College of Physicians; Member of the Association of Military Surgeons of the United States; Member of the American Medical Association.

FRANK DAMAZO, M.D.

Doctor Frank Damazo was born on 11 November 1923, in New Bedford, Massachusetts, the fourth of ten children of immigrant parents from the Portuguese Azore Islands. Doctor Damazo received his medical degree from Loma Linda University School of Medicine, Loma Linda, California, in 1948. He completed an internship at Maumee Valley Hospital in Toledo, Ohio in 1949, and a one year surgical residency at the same hospital in 1950.

A short time in private practice in Maine (1950–51) was followed by two years (1951–53) in the Medical Corps of the United States Army, with service in Korea. Doctor Damazo then completed a surgical residency at Henry Ford Hospital in Detroit, Michigan (1953–56). Since that time he has been in surgical practice in Frederick, Maryland.

Doctor Damazo is a Diplomate of the American Board of Surgery; a Diplomate of the American Board of Abdominal Surgery, and a Fellow of the American College of Surgeons.

CHAPLAIN THOMAS A. GREEN

Chaplain Tom Green was born on 1 June 1927 in Ventor, New Jersey. He was baptized into the Seventh-day Adventist church in Hyattsville, Maryland in April 1942. He graduated from the Academy in 1944, and then enrolled in Washington Missionary College, now known as Columbia Union College.

Just after he finished his Freshman year he was drafted into the Army, returning to the college in 1947 to major in theology and history and receive a Bachelor of Arts degree in 1951. In August 1950 at Worcester, Massachusetts, Tom married Priscilla Mae Littlefield.

Tom began denominational employment as a bindery worker in the Review and Herald Publishing Association in June 1943 and continued this part-time employment until drafted into the United States Army in July 1945. From July 1945 until November 1946, Tom was trained and utilized as a surgical technician by the Army. During this period of military service, he was stationed at Camp Crowder, Missouri; Fitzsimmons General Hospital, Denver, Colorado; and Oliver General Hospital, Augusta, Georgia.

He was accepted in June 1951 as a ministerial intern in the New Jersey Conference of Seventh-day Adventists. In July 1956, at the annual Camp Meeting in Kingston, New Jersey, Tom was ordained to the ministry. He continued as a pastor in the New Jersey Conference until November 1961, when he became a civilian chaplain of the Adventist Church in the Washington, D.C. area. This role continued until May 1974. He took an active role in the development of the concept, site choice, and architectural plans and building of the Washington Adventist Servicemen's Center. Tom served as the Center's director during the entire period of its existence from February 1968 until it ceased all operations in May 1974.

With the closing of the Servicemen's Center, Tom accepted the invitation to be an associate chaplain of the Porter Memorial Hospital in Denver, Colorado, beginning 1 June 1974. The abilities and personality which made him a successful civilian chaplain in the military community, and the experience gained in that ministry, doubtless helped him to be an effective witness in his continuing work as a hospital chaplain.

Tom was certified in 1976 as a Fellow in the College of Chaplains of the American Protestant Hospital Association. He continued to serve as a chaplain at Porter Memorial Hospital in Denver until his retirement in January 1990.

APPENDIX B

FACT SHEET

For Volunteer Candidates at Fort Sam Houston, Texas

PROJECT WHITECOAT

Project WHITECOAT is the official designation of the volunteer program conducted by the US Army Medical Research Institute of Infectious Diseases. This program originated in 1954 following a series of meetings between representatives of the General Conference of the Seventh-day Adventist Church and of the Surgeon General of the Army. The individuals most closely associated with this phase of the program were Elder W. R. Beach, Secretary of the General Conference, and Brigadier General W.D. Tigertt, MC, who, at that time as a colonel, was Chief of the Special Operations Branch, Walter Reed Army Institute of Research (WRAIR), Washington, D.C.

Project WHITECOAT was established originally to determine the vulnerability of man to attack with biological weapons using Q fever as a prototype. At that time the program was an integral part of WRAIR, and all volunteer studies were conducted by the Walter Reed component at Fort Detrick. Colonel Tigertt was designated by the Sec-

retary of the Army as the person responsible for all volunteer participation in this multifaceted research project.

On 20 June 1956 the US Army Medical Unit, Fort Detrick was activated by WRAMC General Order No. 37 under command of Colonel W.D. Tigertt. With activation of this unit, responsibility for Project WHITECOAT was transferred from Walter Reed Army Institute of Research to the US Army Medical Unit, where it has remained to date. The name of the US Army Medical Unit was changed in January 1969 to the US Army Medical Research Institute of Infectious Disease (USAMRIID).

Personnel for Project WHITECOAT are recruited from military personnel with a 1–A–O (conscientious objector) classification undergoing Basic and Advanced Individual Training at The Medical Training Center, Fort Sam Houston. Twice a year, the Commanding Officer and the Detachment Commander, USAMRIID and the Director of the National Service Organization of the Seventh-day Adventist General Conference interview personnel at the Medical Training Center considered eligible for Project WHITECOAT. They are given a complete and comprehensive explanation of the program including discussion of the risk involved. The following day they are interviewed individually and offered an additional opportunity to ask questions. At that time they may indicate their desire to participate in Project WHITECOAT. The number of individuals volunteering for this program is generally much larger than the number that can be accepted. Selection is based on suitability of the volunteer for this particular assignment and the needs of USAMRIID.

Those selected are assigned to the Institute specifically for participation in Project WHITECOAT. Immediately upon arrival each WHITECOAT member undergoes a thorough medical examination. This includes a complete history, a detailed physical examination and extensive laboratory studies. Occasionally some abnormality may disqualify him from participation in a research study.

After administrative processing they are assigned to various noncombatant type duties such as medical laboratory technician, medical corpsman, medical supply clerk, medical maintenance technician, animal caretaker, etc. WHITECOAT personnel generally remain at USAMRIID during the remainder of their military service obligation. These individuals are full time soldiers and receive no special consideration for participating in volunteer studies.

When a research study in volunteers is to be conducted, the required number of WHITECOAT personnel are given a comprehensive briefing by the Commanding Officer as to the purpose and nature of the project, the risk involved, and exactly what is expected of the par-

ticipant. After answering any questions that might arise, each subject is interviewed individually, given an additional opportunity to ask questions, and then indicates his desires as to participation in that particular study. If he volunteers he is required to sign the standard consent form. When an individual indicates that he would prefer not to participate in a particular study it usually is for personal reasons such as his wife having a baby, he is to be best man at his sister's wedding, or some similar reason.

Immediately upon admission to the research ward each volunteer undergoes a thorough medical evaluation to assure that he has not developed some condition that would contraindicate participation in the study

The present research program of USAMRIID is completely unclassified and the results, if appropriate, are published in the medical literature. The results of studies in which WHITECOAT volunteers participate are included in these publications.

APPENDIX C

MRVS RECRUITMENT PROCEDURES

One of the mission objectives of the U. S. army Medical Research Institute of Infectious Diseases (USAMRIID) is to develop therapy and preventive measures for naturally occurring high hazard diseases. Since 1975 USAMRIID has conducted human volunteer studies for vaccines and antimalarial and antiviral drugs. Such studies are conducted only after extensive preclinical testing of the vaccine or drug. These human volunteer studies follow the requirements set forth in Department of Defense Directive 3216.2, which establishes policy pertaining to the protection of human volunteers in DoD supported research. Additionally, U. S. Army Regulation, AR 70–25, implements this directive and provides for the following:

1. Protection, to the maximum extent possible, of the fundamental rights and welfare of human volunteers. This protection is meant to encompass basic respect for human dignity and to protect volunteers from harm.

2. Ensure that volunteers are fully informed and voluntarily agree to participate in the research study (informed consent).

USAMRIID recruits Medical Research Volunteers Subjects (MRVS) from Army active duty soldiers in the 232nd Medical Battalion, Academy of Health Sciences, Fort Sam Houston, Texas. The USAMRIID Sergeant Major provides to the soldiers of this battalion a brief orientation describing the mission of the U. S. Army Medical

Research and Development Command (USAMRDC) and USAMRIID and the purpose of recruiting soldiers as MRVS. If the protocol is accepted by this committee, it is then reviewed by the USAMRIID Human Use Committee with specific attention to the following questions:

1. Are the risks of the study outweighed by the benefit to the individual or mankind sufficient enough to justify the volunteer accepting those risks?

2. Are the known or potential risks minimized to the maximum degree possible?

3. Are any residual risks accurately and completely communicated to the volunteer in the informed consent statement and volunteer agreement?

4. Are adequate provisions taken to assure that the rights and welfare of the volunteer will be upheld? These provisions include Privacy Act laws, rights of volunteers to make claims against the government, disability and assurance of required medical care in the event of a trial-associated injury.

5. Will the conduct of the study be monitored by qualified medical and scientific personnel and will the Human Use Committee receive timely reports and follow-up?

The Human Use Committee is composed primarily of individuals who are not affiliated with USAMRIID. Only the chairperson and a MRVS representative are from USAMRIID. The remaining members include the Post chaplain, the Post JAG officer, three civilian scientists, and a civically-active housewife. In addition to conducting the review of all studies involving human volunteers, the USAMRIID Human Use Committee monitors the recruitment of active duty Army soldiers who are interested in volunteering and are then given an in depth briefing lasting approximately ninety minutes. This includes a description of:

1. The voluntary nature of the assignment and of protocol participation.

2. The scientific and human use review processes for protocols.

3. "Life as a MRVS" as described by a soldier currently participating in the volunteer program.

Following this briefing, those soldiers who are interested complete a questionnaire, enclosure 1, and each is interviewed individually. Approximately one third of the soldiers who are interviewed are selected to participate as volunteers. The list of selectees is then given to Personnel Command, Department of the Army, who make the final assignment of the individual soldier based on the current needs of the Army. Once a soldier is recruited, he or she may change their mind about being assigned to USAMRIID any time up to their arrival at Fort Detrick and thereafter may voluntarily withdraw from the MRVS program at any time.

All vaccines or drugs must first go through extensive preclinical testing in accordance with the Food and Drug Administration's Good Laboratory Practices requirements before being considered for testing in human volunteers. The actual protocol for a human study is thoroughly reviewed by the USAMRIID Scientific Review Committee which is composed of scientists and soldiers for the MRVS program.

After the USAMRIID Human Use Committee reviews the study and formulates recommendations, the USAMRIID Commander reviews the protocol and recommendations and either approves or disapproves the study. If the committee disapproves the study, their decision can not be overturned by the Commander. If the Commander approves the protocol, it is then sent to the Human Use Review Office (HURO) for review and approval by the Army Surgeon's General Human Subjects Research Review Board. Before any drug or vaccine can be administered to human volunteers, it must have Food and Drug Administration approval.

Once the protocol involving human volunteers is approved, the MRVS are asked to volunteer for the protocol. Each volunteer is thoroughly informed of the protocol and advised of the possible risks involved. Any questions that he or she may have are answered and points of clarification are made. The volunteer then reads the consent form, enclosure 2, and signs his or her name. At any time before the start of the protocol or during the protocol, the volunteer may withdraw from the program without fear of penalty or reprisal.